The Best **ORAL SEX** Ever

His Guide to Going Down

The Best ORAL SEX Ever

His Guide to Going Down

Yvonne K. Fulbright, PhD

Adams Media
New York London Toronto Sydney New Delhi

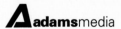

Adams Media
An Imprint of Simon & Schuster, Inc.
100 Technology Center Drive
Stoughton, MA 02072

For information about special discounts for bulk purchases, please contact Simon & Schuster Special Sales at 1-866-506-1949 or business@simonandschuster.com.

The Simon & Schuster Speakers Bureau can bring authors to your live event. For more information or to book an event contact the Simon & Schuster Speakers Bureau at 1-866-248-3049 or visit our website at www.simonspeakers.com.

Interior illustrations © Eric Andrews

Interior photographs © FotoSearch/Image Source

Manufactured in the United States of America

15 2022

Library of Congress Cataloging-in-Publication Data has been applied for.

ISBN 978-1-4405-1080-9
ISBN 978-1-4405-1136-3 (ebook)

To all of my dedicated readers—your interest and enthusiasm in all of my work mean so much!

ACKNOWLEDGMENTS

Thanks to Victoria Sandbrook and Katrina Schroeder, and everyone else on the Adams Media team, for their guidance and feedback. It's always a pleasure to write books for you guys!

My deepest thanks to my amazing family and friends for their never-ending support and encouragement in all that I do: Charles G. Fulbright, Ósk Lárusdóttir Fulbright, Xavier Þór Fulbright, Lauren Fulbright, Rick Barth, Solveig Bergh, Lymaraina D'Souza, Sean Duffy, Tiffany J. Franklin, Bianca A. Grimaldi, Cheri Heathscott, Marci Hunn, Jennifer Kilgus, and Ásgeir Sigfússon—plus everyone at home in Iceland! It has been a breathtaking year of travel, opportunity, growth, and change—and I couldn't have done it without you. xoxo

Contents

INTRODUCTION

Open Up and Say "Ahhhh"

If you've cracked open this book, then your curiosity has been piqued. Oral sex has a way of doing that, beckoning lovers to come get a taste of *this*. Those who have been there know it's *the* means to better, higher peaking. Those who haven't been there and those who've been disappointed by earlier attempts know its reputation for inviting sexual release as nothing else can. They hunger for their fill of the same. There's no doubt that going down on her (and him) has taken center stage in the quest for sexual fulfillment. Seems everyone wants more than a mouthful, and who can blame them?

With oral sex a main mode of climax, including multiple orgasms, for lovers, its role in and influence on a sexual relationship is critical. With the perfect mix of having the right person, in the right moment, with all of the right moves, stellar oral sex can make for some of the most memorable "sexperiences" around. And even when circumstances are a little less than ideal, oral action can still invite some of the hottest sexual exchanges to be had—that's how powerful and pleasure-filled the oral act is in and of itself!

No matter what your sexual exchange, becoming an oral connoisseur is where it's at when it comes to reaching new, literally jaw-dropping sexual heights. The challenge for many, however, revolves around how to make oral sex a fine dining experience for both giver and receiver. While your aim is to make giving head the best ever for *her*, this book is very much about how to make your experience as the giver the best for *you* too. A pleasure shared is a pleasure doubled, after all. Your ability to not only deliver the most effective techniques around, but to love what you're doing and to totally get into the moment is critical to making her erotic experience the ultimate-ever-had grade.

This book is intended for lovers looking for erotic ideas, couples hoping to deal with their oral sex issues, and individuals seeking to make oral sex on her more palpable or more of a priority in their passion pursuits. Meant for adults of all ages, it's for those of you who need and want to know the information vital to realizing yours—and her—maximum pleasure potential via what is affectionately referred to as *cunnilingus* in anything from textbooks to your sex Bible *Cosmopolitan*. Plus, it answers all of those questions that lovers are too afraid or embarrassed to ask, unless they work up the nerve to email a sexologist, like myself, for advice. After years of helping people as a sex educator and relationship expert, I know well the trials and tribulations lovers grapple with when it comes to oral sex. Those coming to me for "confessional" have told me shamelessly or shyly that they adore oral sex, they'd love more oral sex, and that they'll never get enough of it. Talk about sexual appetites!

As with any sex act, oral sex mastery comes with time, dedication, practice, and desire. This book sends you well on your way, offering tips and techniques for your oral pleasures, and strategies for barriers that stand in your way. Upon reading *The Best Oral Sex Ever: His Guide to Going Down*, you'll stand to come away with:

- A whole new level of "sexpertise" when it comes to understanding one of her favorite sex acts, as well as other forms of pleasuring
- Realistic erotic expectations

- Better sex communications skills in letting your needs, concerns, and questions be known
- The information and skills needed to take care of your sexual health and hers while doing what you'll do best
- Tons of instruction for your erotic arsenal on eroticizing oral sex and realizing orgasm, including her potential for multiple orgasms
- Referrals you can turn to for more information

It can't be said enough: Going down on her can offer lovers some of the greatest pleasures and most intimate moments to be had as sexual beings. The experience of launching her into an oral orgasmic orbit is practically beyond words. So the confidence and power trip that comes in knowing that you're an expert in giving oral is like no other ego boost when it comes to your skills set. By the end of this book, you'll be on top of your game, including your abilities to help her feel more than a little sexually satisfied.

As you read through the following pages, it's important to remember that sexual preferences are as numerous as there are people. How to make oral sex an art form for a particular sexual partner needs to be explored and specially tailored to her wants and likes. Some things may work after one or many tries, while some things may not, while other things may work at another stage in the relationship.

So be sure to approach oral sex just as you would any other meal experience. Try a new venue; sample a different dish; ask that your portion be served up with a twist; add some spices. Then talk about how much you're savoring this carnal cuisine, before sitting back and enjoying all the exquisite eroticism to be had with the tip of the tongue, and then some, for years to come.

Speaking of which, if you're in your current relationship for the long haul, you may want to come back to this book more than once, especially in light of how we all evolve as lovers in our pleasures, reactions, and abilities. How to keep oral intimacy original, red hot, and Eros-inducing needs to be revisited from time to time in keeping the passion alive, with the sweet bit being that it can!

No matter what your quest, it is my hope that this book will make your endeavors all the easier, helping you to see oral sex in a whole new, healthy light. In guiding your "sexplorations" and in giving you all of the information you need, in my sex expert opinion, you'll soon be delivering oral like a sex pro.

CHAPTER 1

Our Intrigue with Oral Sex

Muff diving, eating someone out, going down, poon job . . . . The slang terms and euphemisms for oral sex on a female are very creative, often quite comical, and—in the very least—numerous. They speak volumes as to the obsession we humans have with the mouth going South when fooling around with a partner. Google *oral sex* and 12,300,000 pages come up for that term alone. People around the world are intrigued with the eroticism involved in giving the genitals a slip of the tongue and more. To say we're orally fixated is an understatement.

Just So We're on the Same Page . . .

Performing oral sex is a universal sexual experience enjoyed by millions as a part of foreplay, as a part of afterplay (that lovely, intimate, coming down period following sexual intercourse), or as the main sex event. In those racy trysts involving more than two sexual partners, it can be experienced during sexual intercourse. In any case, oral-genital contact, more commonly known as *oral sex* involves giving or receiving pleasure delivered to a person's sexual organs primarily via the lips and tongue. This is typically done in a rhythmic licking or sucking fashion using one's mouth, though any number of techniques can be employed, as we'll cover in-depth throughout this book.

Cunnilingus, from the Latin *cunnus* (vulva) and *lingere* (to lick), is the technical term for orally stimulating a female's genitals. Action typically focuses on her clitoris, the inner and outer lips, and vaginal opening. *Analingus*, also known as *rimming*, a *rim job*, *ass licking*, *eating ass*, or *tossing salad*, refers to oral-anal contact. Anal-oral sex may be a part of cunnilingus or the sole event of a sex session.

Now while some of the names used for oral sex may sound technical, depending on whom you're talking to, these types of sexual exchanges can be quite titillating. Given that eating her out is a highly effective erotic technique, it has held rapture for humans throughout the ages. The rimming bit—which we'll cover here and there throughout—is more of a, shall we say, acquired taste, but a delectable one for those into it. Whether shared as a sacred act of partner worship, sought for its scintillating sensations, or pursued as a prime opportunity to get down and dirty, any of these oral adventures is the favorite kind of sex to be had for a number of lovers for a number of reasons.

Why She Loves Oral Sex

Many women love receiving oral sex not only because getting the "ultimate kiss" feels incredible, but she has learned that it's critical to her orgasm as well. Some women are only able to climax from having someone go down on them since the clitoris, the hub of women's pleasure, receives so much attention during the oral act. Others need oral sex, and the orgasm from cunnilingus, to reach climax during intercourse. In many cases, a female's orgasm from cunnilingus is fast, relaxing, and healing. It's an aphrodisiac on a psychological level, and this most intimate of sex play often makes women feel desired, respected, and appreciated.

Rolls off the Tongue

"Oral sex is the cream on the cake as far as sexual experiences for me. It makes me cum like nothing else both while my partner is going down on me, then later during intercourse. I have a tough time reaching climax in any other way. But I'm not complaining since, hands down, oral sex from a skilled lover is absolutely divine." } Michelle

Pleasure from Power

The ego trip from the power element alone in getting head can be intoxicating for her. Being the object of a partner's devotion only adds to the adoration she has for oral. With her dream lover between her legs, how can she help but not get caught up in the high of being serviced or pleasured?! She has let someone get up close and personal in her most private space, and that person—you—is going to town, lost in the mission of maximizing her pleasure. This only gets hotter when she glances down at what's going on between her legs. The mere visual stimulation that comes from seeing (and imagining in her off-time) your head bobbing, drunk with desire, can be highly arousing.

Of course, let's not forget the power trip in this exchange for you and the elation that comes along with being the giver. While often cast as the submissive in being the provider, *you're not*. You're actually the partner in charge. In getting the green light to go down, you've been granted VIP access to your partner's prime hot spots. Her pleasuring is in your hands. You control your hottie's sexual destiny (at least for the moment) in commanding the action—all with the best seat in the house.

So take a moment as you're working away to get turned on by seeing your gal become sexually excited, an experience made even sweeter when the object of your affection hits heaven. She may not be in that alone. As giver, you can thrive on your own "mental orgasm" in knowing that she is thoroughly enjoying your efforts. You created the moment necessary for sexual release, and that can be incredibly fulfilling.

Sex Savvy

Despite its mass popularity, believe it or not, oral sex is on the books as illegal in some states, like Indiana. Getting caught engaging in these "acts against nature," even when consensual and with another adult, can mean can getting fined and imprisoned for up to one year in states classifying oral sex as a felony. So for those of you dead set on breaking the law, let this bad-ass bit fuel hotter oral. After all, such restrictions and concerns have helped to fetishize oral sex over the ages and have turned it into a mystical ecstasy of sorts—and all the more desirable. So for those of you who can legally have cunnilingus, stoke the same thrills by pretending you're doing it in Indiana.

Oral Sex Today

Since the sexual revolution of the 1960s and 1970s, the United States has seen a growing acceptance of oral sex. More popular than ever, it is widely practiced today, with the increase in mouth-genital techniques seen as one of the most dramatic changes in marital sex alone in the past fifty years. Whereas a generation ago, oral sex was seen as a shameful taboo, such sex play has become an acceptable behavior. That's not to say, however, that it doesn't still pose controversy. As recently as 2010, dictionaries were removed from southern California classrooms after a parent complained that a child could read the definition for the term *oral sex*. The school district responded by pulling *Merriam Webster's Tenth Edition* from shelves for fear of being too "sexually graphic" and inappropriate for certain age groups. Despite regularly ruffling feathers, oral sex has become regarded more and more as an important and healthy component of one's sexual self.

While not as widely practiced as other types of sexual deeds, oral sex is a very common practice. If any hesitancy you have in engaging in oral comes down to safety in numbers, rest assured. Various studies show that such sexual behaviors are practiced by the majority of people, with about 90 percent of men and women ages 25-44 reporting having engaged in oral sex as givers or receivers!

For that, we should perhaps be thanking the media for plugging oral sex. It's hard not to notice that giving the ultimate in oral sex tips are regular headliners and features in online and hardcopy media outlets alike. This eagerness for anything oral has, however, perpetuated some of the myths and misconceptions tackled in this book. All this attention feeds many of the stereotypes swirling around oral sex when it comes to gender differences. Articles for men tend to detach oral sex for either partner from the emotional side of the relationship; women's articles tend to treat oral sex as something done to enhance relationship intimacy. For him, it's cast as an experience in and of itself, requiring none of the niceties or symbolism it supposedly does for her. While there is some truth in some generalities, buyer beware! In enjoying such articles, you need to be mindful about the messages you're getting, recognizing how the media may be influencing your thoughts, her expectations, and your practices around such pleasuring.

Which Women Are Into It?

A far cry from previous generations, many women today have become enthusiastic about letting men go downtown. A much larger percentage of women under 50, compared to those over 50, have ever given or received oral sex in their lifetime.

Studies involving college women have found that attractive women are much likelier to engage in oral sex and other sexual acts, including woman-on-top position. Researchers believe that this could be because of the expectations these women put on themselves, the more frequent opportunities they have to engage in such sex play, or simply because they feel a sense of sexual power in being beauties. Still, even more recent research has found that the vast majority of women are engaging in some type of oral sex or another, with most young women engaging in these activities because they enjoy them.

Sex Savvy

When it comes to ethnic differences, the National Social Life, Health, and Aging Project found that white women are about 30 percent likelier to give or receive oral sex than are African Americans, with Latinas falling midway between the two groups.

Why Being a Brainiac Is Sexy

Investigations on who has done what orally have revealed that one's education, which is often related to one's social class, is a factor. The majority of people in the United States who don't engage in oral sex are in the lowest educational groups. The higher one's education level, the likelier it is that he or she is engaging in oral sex. Men who don't graduate from high school are less likely to have performed oral sex than men who are better educated.

Women who have attended college are twice as likely to report giving and receiving oral sex than those women who didn't complete high school. Only 41 percent of women with less than high school diplomas have performed oral sex on a man, while only 49 percent have been the recipient of cunnilingus. Compare this to the 80 percent of women with at least some college education who have experienced either.

The women's liberation movement, reproductive rights, and support in exploring their sexuality are among the reasons believed to impact a female's sexual practices to a certain extent. Women engaged in these social movements tend to be more educated and more aware. They also tend to be more accomplished in some ways, like their level of educational attainment. Educated girls, it seems, are more likely to diversify their sexual repertoire between the sheets. No wonder it pays to stay in school!

Sex Q & A

Are humans the only species on earth that engage in oral sex?

No, animals may engage in oral-genital stimulation, especially when the female is in *estrue* (heat). During this rare time of year, a male may lick her genitals in response to pheromones she's giving off.

Oral Sex and Intimacy

Oral sex can be a very personal, intimate sexual experience for some people and no big deal to others. For some people, oral exchanges are reserved for partners whom they feel really close to. They may regard oral intimacies as a marker of how lovers feel about each other sexually and emotionally, making a relationship all the more exclusive. For others, it's a staple part of every sexual affair, a cheap thrill handled with indifference. In a number of cases, the degree of intimacy can come down to the situation and with whom you're exchanging lip service.

Casual or not, having oral sex is quite physically intimate for both the giver and receiver. In most giving scenarios, your face is nestled in your partner's loins, your lips, tongue, and face pressed against the softness of her thighs. No matter the social meaning of this act, being up close and personal can make any experience extremely emotionally intimate. You can hardly get any more physically personal than involving your head and face in pleasuring your lover. Add to that the symbolism involved, and it can be a huge deal.

Symbolically, oral sex is the meeting of the cultured, reasoning, intellectual (top) half of one's self with what's regarded as another's raw, carnal, unrefined smut central. The impermissible nature of this meeting violates social order. It's seen as a "corruption" of the self, even in the most celebratory of sensually fused circumstances. A sense of intimacy—and libidinal energy—is practically immediate in lovers daring to defy social taboos together. Casts Romeo and Juliet longings in a whole new light, no?

The Importance of Oral Sex

Regardless of the type of relationship you're in (or not), or the circumstances around your carnal encounter, oral sex has come to mean hot sex. Because it is a self-esteem booster to get some or give some, oral sex can make or break a specific sex session. It can heavily influence the quality of a couple's sex life for the better when regularly engaged in, or for the worse when given zero attention. This very intimate form of connection can be a relationship strengthener. In *The Hite Report*, women reported that a lover going down on them implied a special kind of acceptance. It was meaningful for a partner to put his mouth down there and to go exploring. Oral sex was seen as being the closest two people can get physically and resulted in positive feelings for her sense of femaleness.

Oral sex is the best kind of sex for some people, with many holding that it is unlike anything else. This sexy gift of pleasure offers excitement, variety, exhilaration, and closeness. Sex partners adore the more precise targeting of erogenous zones that comes with oral sex, often feeling heightened sensitivity as a lover makes them moan. A lover's tongue and lips feel amazing in being soft, moist, and warm against the sensitive genitals. Whether giving or receiving, oral sex can be meditative, with either partner slipping into a zen-like state of enlightenment in reaching a heightened state of awareness that can be spiritual in nature.

Rolls Off the Tongue

"One of my most treasured moments was when my boyfriend and I had sex for the first time. It wasn't the significance of it being the 'first' that stands out so much as that he went down on me both before and after intercourse. He really wanted to make sure that I was sexually satisfied, and had no qualms about what it would take to make me multiorgasmic, including going down there after we'd worked up a sweat!" }Signe

CHAPTER 2

Sexual Anatomy: Passion-Inducing Parts

You know that her private parts entail a vulva and vagina, but do you really know which exact parts are best when getting more than a little bit fresh? Her groin is covered with hidden treasures just begging to be unearthed, aching to be probed by the tip of your tongue. Whether bringing her response to life or maximizing her pleasure once the juices are flowing, you'll want to spend some time becoming well acquainted with her oft-overlooked, but most reactive hot spots. Prepare to see her wares in a whole new light.

| Mapping Her Landscape

While some people are lucky enough to cover the anatomy of sex at some point in their schooling, the vast majority never thoroughly learn about the ins and outs of some of our most amazing private parts! The result: Many lovers have no clue what is where, how to play with a juicy bit, or how to reach peak sexual response with spots that are solely for pleasure. Not your average biology lesson, the following sections on her genitalia are among the most important in this book if your aim is to become a better, savvier lover. Here, you get the quick 'n' dirty down-low on sexual makeup for planning your carnal connect-the-dots.

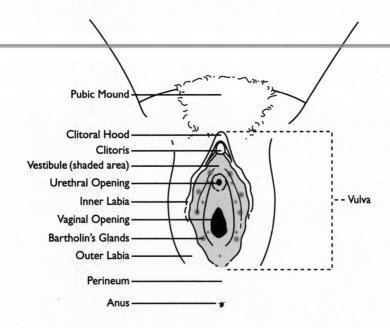

Pubic Mound

Clitoral Hood
Clitoris
Vestibule (shaded area)
Urethral Opening
Inner Labia
Vaginal Opening
Bartholin's Glands
Outer Labia

Perineum

Anus

Vulva

Her External Genitalia

Known collectively as the *vulva* (or pudendum), a female's external genitals consist of the following:

- **Mons pubis.** Also known as the *mons veneris*, this pad of tissue rests atop a female's pubic bone and, in its natural state, is covered with pubic hair once she hits puberty. The purpose of the mons pubis, it is speculated, is to bear the brunt of sexual thrusting, protecting a woman's pubic bone.

- **Outer lips.** Also called the *labia majora*, these rounded, sensitive skin folds are covered with pubic hair and contain glands that produce her unique scent. They serve to protect her inner vulva.

- **Inner lips.** Sometimes referred to as the *labia minora*, these often thinner and smoother folds of skin are found between her outer lips and the vaginal entrance that join at the top of the clitoris to form the clitoral hood. They may or may not be longer or more pronounced than the outer lips. Full of nerve endings, these lips may be pink, bright red, or deep brown to black. They are often damp since their sebaceous glands produce a *sebum* (a lubricant) which coats the skin to form a waterproof, protective covering when combined with secretions from the vagina. Together, the inner and outer lips are known collectively as the *labia*. Both sets of lips are highly erogenous.

- **Clitoris.** The hub of her sexual pleasuring and orgasm, this most sensitive sexual organ—cradled between her labia—houses about 8,000 nerve endings. Extending anywhere from two to four centimeters on the outside of the body, the clitoris actually continues internally back into her reproductive system. Composed of a *clitoral glans* (head), where the inner and outer lips meet, its body contains spongy erectile tissue that fills with blood when she becomes excited. This tissue involves a pair of *corpora cavernosa* (two clitoral shafts) which extend back into the body, wrapping around her vaginal opening, urethra, urethral sponge, and vagina. These *legs* or *crura* can be as long as nine centimeters.

- **Clitoral hood.** This sheath of tissue (also known as the *prepuce*) protects the clitoris along with the *commissure* (an area of skin which can be viewed by gently pulling back on the outer lips and hood). Its purpose is to protect her crown jewel from becoming over-stimulated.
- **Urethral opening.** Often mistaken for the clitoris, this protrusion, through which urine passes, is found between her clitoris and vaginal opening. A few women find it stimulating to have this area played with.
- **Vaginal opening.** Typically one inch in diameter, the *introitus* (as it's also known) opens to the vaginal canal.
- **Perineum.** This soft tissue between the vaginal opening and anus contains nerve endings and spongy erectile tissue. It is the area where much of her pelvic floor muscles criss-cross each other.
- **Bartholin's glands.** These are located on either side of the vaginal opening and provide lubrication during sexual response, secreting a small amount of fluid.

Rolls Off the Tongue

"One of the most touching moments I've ever had during oral was when my lover went down on me for the first time. He delicately played with my clit, as though testing the waters before pulling back to just look at my vulva, then exclaiming, 'You're beautiful!' It was so sweet." }

Michaela

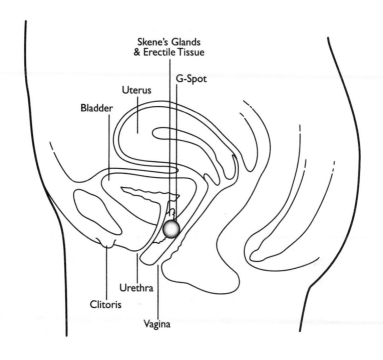

Skene's Glands
& Erectile Tissue

G-Spot

Uterus

Bladder

Urethra

Clitoris

Vagina

Her Internal Genitalia

A female's internal reproductive system consists of the ovaries, fallopian tubes, uterus, cervix, and vagina, but here, we focus on the parts that you may choose to stimulate during oral sex.

- **Vagina:** A highly muscular organ connecting the vaginal opening and cervix, the vaginal canal sits at a 45-degree angle, extending four inches deep in a female's unaroused state. With sexual excitement, this elastic canal can double in depth and width. Its greatest concentration of nerves is in its lower one-third.
- **Cervix:** The small, fleshy dome-like opening to the uterus, the cervix is a hot spot for some. Pressure or thrusting against the

cervix can, however, be uncomfortable or painful for a number of women.

- **G-spot:** A nickname for the *Gräfenberg spot*, this female prostate or urethral sponge, as it's also known, is located approximately two inches up the front (abomdinal side) wall of the vaginal canal. Made up of paraurethral glands, ducts, and blood vessels, this tissue swells during sexual arousal, with its erogenous reactions varying from woman to woman.

Sex Savvy

Oh, oh, oh! The three o's—oral, orgasm, and oxytocin—make for a killer combination. During orgasm, the body releases hormones thought to be associated with attachment, bonding, and closeness: vasopressin and oxytocin, your "cuddle chemicals." The neurohormone oxytocin spikes three to five times higher than its normal levels in a female's bloodstream, brain, and spinal cord just before climax. In both sexes, this reaction sensitizes skin, encouraging more touch. Be sure to capitalize on this information!

What Happens When She Gets Hot and Horny

First researched and outlined by sexologists in the 1960s, the "sexual response cycle" involves a general pattern of events that a number of people typically go through when sexually stimulated. This model for understanding the process of getting all hot and bothered is largely seen as having five phases:

- Desire
- Arousal

- Plateau
- Orgasm
- Resolution

While these stages generally happen in sequence, your lover can experience these responses in any order. She may also "stray" off of this beaten path, with her body doing what works for her. There is nothing wrong with this. The blueprint for sexual response varies from person to person and from time to time, and is influenced by a number of factors.

Many researchers, in fact, are saying that the original linear sexual response cycle doesn't work for women, since many of them don't move progressively or sequentially through those stages. Conversely, some may not even experience all stages, jumping from arousal to orgasm and satisfaction. Or they may experience climax, but no sexual desire. Though they're also often cast as "abnormal" if they don't respond in a certain way, men and women who don't conform to the cycle's patterns can still fully partake in pleasurable sexual experiences.

Other circular models, involving factors like seduction or emotional intimacy, have been proposed in trying to capture the female sexual response. It's simply important that you know the potential differences between your sexual response cycle and hers.

With that said, let's look at one of the major ways sexual response has been captured by sex researchers.

Desire

An entity of its own, separate from sexual arousal, desire motivates us to get sexually active. Desire can be sparked—intentionally or not—by sex objects, physical arousal, fantasies, spontaneous excitement, longings, images, sounds, scents, memories, interests, or experiences—any of which can be sensual, pornographic, thrilling, or heart-soaring.

Desire can come on unexpectedly or you may actively seek to feel consumed with its libidinal urging. In propelling our sex drive, desire urges us to seek out a partner, pursue sexual opportunities, engage in sexual behaviors, and realize sexual satisfaction. It is impacted by our health, mood, and attitudes, among a whole host of biological, psychological, social, and relational factors.

Sex Savvy

Does desire really come before arousal or is it the other way around? Research is suggesting that desire may not necessarily lead to sexual excitement, but that it may be a type of afterthought. Desire may be a reaction we have to a subliminal or physical sensation, like touch. In other words, your body and hers appear to be primed for sex!

Arousal

During the Excitement Phase, your body is preparing itself for sex. Whether it's you or your partner, you may notice faster, heavier breathing, an accelerated heart rate, a sex flush (typically a reddening of the chest and/or face) or lubrication. This is in large part because the body is experiencing *myotonia* (muscle tension) and *vasocongestion* (the accumulation of blood in the genitals, which causes them to become darker, more swollen, and harder). As your lover's body gets ready to make contact with yours, natural lubrication pushes its way through her vaginal walls. The Bartholin's glands, too, begin secreting lubricating fluids. Her uterus may elevate slightly, and her vagina may ache. Her clitoris swells with blood, the erectile tissue becomes erect and even doubles in size. Her vaginal lips may be more visible and firm. Her breasts may swell and enlarge, with her nipples possibly becoming hard and erect.

Plateau

A state of high arousal, the Plateau Phase extends heightened sexual response with continued sex flush, faster breathing, and a higher blood pressure and heart rate. Some may even experience short muscle spasms in their face, hands, and feet. During this time, a woman's incredibly sensitive clitoris is fully erect, pulling back up under her clitoral hood. Her sex skin has become its darkest on her inner and outer lips, areola, and nipples. Her vagina continues to lengthen as her uterus lifts up off of the vaginal canal and her vaginal entrance tightens. She's becoming ever more lubricated.

Orgasm

This peak of sexual arousal physiologically involves an intense series of rhythmic pelvic contractions as the body releases sexual tension, muscles contracting. One's pulse rate, breathing, blood pressure, and sex flush are at their highest levels. But that's just one way to describe her climax. Ask a gal how she would describe an orgasm, and you can get any number of incredible responses, like "pure energy," "light," "heaven," "awesome," and "indescribable."

Sex Q & A

Is orgasm necessary for sexual satisfaction?

While climax is often seen as the *crème de la crème* of sexual response, it isn't vital to sexual gratification. A number of men and women have reported that sex without orgasm can be very satisfying. This is in part because they value the other oh-so-sexy components involved in ideal sex, including being in-sync with their partners, erotic intimacy, connectedness, and being present and uninhibited.

In some cases, female ejaculation may accompany climax. Most often due to G-spot stimulation, this is the emission of a prostatic-like fluid known as *ambrosia*, which can be secreted during climax. It's released mostly via her urethra, but is *not* urine. This perfectly natural sexual release can happen each time a gal experiences a lot of sexual excitement, sometimes, or never.

Resolution

In this final phase of the sexual response cycle, lovers come down from heightened arousal. As blood pressure drops and one's heart rate and breathing slow, the sex flush disappears, and blood drains out of the pelvis. Your lover will come down from her orgasmic platform gradually, with her breasts becoming their regular size, her clitoris resuming its normal position, her uterus shrinking, and her vagina relaxing.

While it's great to have a solid understanding of human sexual response, whether it's yours or your lover's, remember that this is a loose road map for a lot of people, but not everyone, every time. So don't get hung up on what's going on (or not). Get caught up in what's going on in the moment, the sexual energy exchange, and the fun to be had in pursuing a shared pleasure, as all of that is what puts everything over the top.

Sex Savvy

Stephen Taylor of the U.K. holds the Guinness World Record for longest tongue, measuring at 3.74 inches beyond the center of his closed top lip.

| Meet Your Tongue

It's all too easy to dive into what's below-the-belt in charting your sexual pleasure pursuits. But when it comes to oral sex, it's not a bad idea to examine the muscular organ of the mouth in addition to the pelvic area's playground. Your tongue can very well be considered a sexual organ in its own right. It's not only one of the main sources of exhilaration for a receiver, but this body part plays a major role in a giver's pleasuring as well, and in ways that are often neglected. So let's explore the love muscle that will bring your lover's gems to life.

The tongue is a mass of muscles, glands, and fat that enhances oral sex via:

- **Movement.** The tongue can move in almost every direction, as well as compress and expand. It enables you to manipulate the genitals with up-down, side to side, and in and out motions, and with great skill and exact pressure.
- **Texture.** Coated with a moist, pink tissue known as mucosa, the tongue is covered with tiny bumps called papillae which give it its rough texture. These are what create the friction that adds to the sensations you deliver.
- **Taste.** The papillae are covered with thousands of taste buds, which are collections of nerve-like cells that connect to the brain via nerve pathways. Each contains 50 to 150 taste receptor cells for detecting the chemical makeup of solutions, enabling you to detect if your lover's genitals or fluids are sweet, salty, bitter, sour (acid), umami (savory), and fatty. The flavor of your feast is a combination of taste, smell, touch, temperature, and consistency (texture).
- **Feel.** Your tongue is sensitive to thermal and tactile sensations, helping you to analyze all of those other qualities that add to your pleasures, like the groin's density, oiliness, texture, and viscosity (consistency).
- **Moisture.** The tongue is covered by a double-layered mucous membrane, the *epithelial* (surface) layer of which secretes mucus to moisten your mouth and whatever you're munching on.

It may seem a little silly to point out these characteristics until you consider just how little attention these qualities of the tongue are given. While food and wine connoisseurs give a great deal of thought to their palate—and what's going on in the mouth—even the best of oral sex enthusiasts don't give a second thought to what their tongue is truly experiencing beyond initial taste and texture perceptions. Yet tuning into the texture, taste, feel, and moisture components of giving and receiving oral sex can heighten the eroticism involved, putting lovers fully in tune with their sexual responses and the sex act itself. Don't deprive yourself of experiencing oral to its fullest!

Rolls Off the Tongue

"It's so easy to get caught up in what I'm doing, namely technique, when I provide pleasuring. But when you tune into what your tongue is experiencing, you start to notice subtleties in the action—and reactions I'm having—which makes for a richer, and tastier, experience." } Jeff

CHAPTER 3

Naked Twister Gets Naughty: Positions for Oral Sex

Naked Twister takes on totally new meaning when you approach traditional sexual positions with oral sex in mind. How you lay, stand, bend, and angle your bodies influences the sensations you deliver and how easily she can relish the sensations meant solely for her. While some positions are ideal for peak performance, others are pursued simply for the variety, for shaking up your routine, while others are meant to amp up excitement in their novelty or exotic nature. Bottom line: she's still getting oral (and loving it) and the mere adventure of strategizing positions and building your sexual repertoire can be the components that make your next "sexchange" absolutely fantastic.

Note: some of these positions may require a great deal of athleticism, strength, and/or flexibility. Realize that not everyone is cut out for every sexual position. While exciting and enticing, don't push the limits on what you or your partner is capable of, as it's anything but sexy to wind up in the ER with an injury!

Rolls Off the Tongue

"After being in a *long* relationship, it's important to mix things up so it doesn't seem mundane and keeps things interesting. New stuff, variety, keeps the passion rolling." } Brent

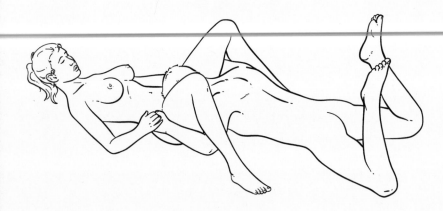

| The Classic

Why couples love it: This relaxing, comfortable position offers you all access to her groin, making any penetration of her anus easy, as well, if that's just what the doctor ordered. The classic also allows for a strong, upward stroking motion with the more textured top surface of your tongue.

Her: The classic takes a load off as she gets to lay back and relax as you go to town. Having her propped up on pillows is optional and quite ideal in helping her to visually enjoy your Oscar performance.

You: While you can kneel between your lover's thighs, it's easier to lie down on your stomach, your arms wrapped under her legs for better leverage, support, control, and stimulation. Another way to approach her is by lying down in a position perpendicular to her body. This position also reduces stress on your neck.

Variations:

- Try raising one or both of her legs over your shoulder(s).
- Bend either or both of her legs into her chest.
- Prop her feet on your shoulders.
- Have her legs splayed or close together.
- Instead of facing her, position yourself so that you're looking the other way.
- Hold one of her legs up for easier access to her vulva and more direct clitoral stimulation.
- Sit on her chest for an almost 69.
- For more direct anal play, have her lift her legs completely over your head.
- Scoot her to the edge of the bed so that her legs dangle over the side.

Tips:

- Place a pillow under her bum for a better angle and greater comfort.
- Grasp and lift her butt as you cast your spells.
- Take action off the bed, trying other flat surfaces for the classic, like your back yard or sofa.
- Gently push upward on her lower stomach with your hand, as this stretches her skin away from her pubic bone, heightening sensations.

- Sit on her legs for a nice I'm-in-charge, pin down effect.
- Encourage her to move, especially in helping you to hit the right spot.
- Sit at the edge of a sofa with her lying on the floor in front of you. Now place her legs on either side of you, which forces her pelvis to tilt upward. Lean forward to enjoy.

Starfish

Why couples love it: Anything exotic is automatically sexy.

Her: Have her on her back, legs and arms spread (and perhaps gently bound to the bedposts, hmmm?).

You: You're lying on your stomach, positioned diagonally across her body so that your head can tuck between her legs.

Tip: "Torture" her by keeping her legs spread while the action becomes more heated. Do this by pressing down on the knees or calves and playing with the back of the knees or the sexual reflexology point San-Yin-Chiao. This point, where the three energy channels intersect, is inside of the shin, approximately three inches above the anklebone and beside the shinbone. Press it to stimulate a major love point of the legs.

If you're into it, ask her to use a free, well lubricated hand to play with your perineum or anus. Just don't lose your concentration.

On Your Knees (a.k.a. Standing)

Why couples love it: Who doesn't like it when somebody looks like they're begging to attend to your every oral need?? It plays into one's, at least occasional, desire to be dominant. For both lovers, this position is great for those after a quickie, especially in public places!

Her: She may want to lean against a firm support, like a couch or wall, not only for comfort, but for better balance as well.

You: Kneel in front of your lover, resting your knees on a pillow, cushion, or blanket so that this position isn't too hard on your knees.

Tip: Grip her hips and bum. In pleasuring her, this helps you to dig into her vulva with a bit more force. Consider seducing her with this move the next time you undress her!

Variations:

- Have her prop one of her legs up on a support for greater control as she stands.
- Place one of her legs over your shoulder. (To help her maintain her balance, place an arm around her opposite thigh, supporting the small of her lower back with your hand.)
- Have her face away from you and stick out her butt for better coming from behind access.
- Sit between and under her legs.
- She can also totally bend over to show off her full moon for even greater access.

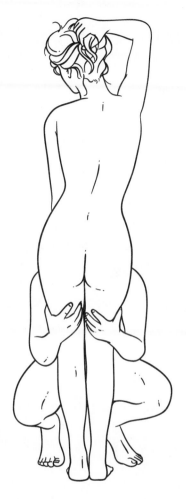

| Sitting

Why couples love it: So many sitting surfaces of various heights to choose from! Plus, it can be easier on your neck and she can open her legs W-I-D-E. She loves that she gets to see you between her legs and that it's easy for you to practice so many strokes.

Her: She sits in the chair of choice (e.g., barstool, armchair, stool, recliner, or kitchen table chair) and is to hook her ankles around the front two legs or over the arms for easier access.

You: Her height on the chair (plus the length of your own body) will determine if you need to go at this one sitting on the floor, on your knees, squatting, or standing.

Variations: Don't limit yourself to traditional chairs. Think anywhere anyone can sit, like your dining room table, kitchen counter, the stairs, the edge of the bed, or your car's back seat. Up for a real challenge? Have her assume a squatting position.

Tips:

- Ask her to show some appreciation for the undying hero worship by delivering a loving, killer head massage as you work away.
- She can also cup the back of your head to encourage more vigorous or deeper action when desired, if that's guidance you'd like.
- Have her sit in a swivel chair to better direct your movements.

| Face-Sitting

Why couples love it: As rider, she takes charge, sliding across your tongue and mouth. This is ideal for those wanting direct oral contact with the genitals and anus. She's going to adore it for being able to control your speed, pressure, and the angle of her pelvis, directing where she wants more stimulation. With you under her, she can also drift off into her own world, which may help her climax.

Her: She's to straddle you, placing her knees on either side of your chest before sitting on it. To make this position as comfortable as possible, have her lean forward. Remind her that she can lower her body for more pressure or elevate herself more for less stimulation.

You: You're on your back. You just need to move your head, mouth, and tongue, allowing yourself to get into it and letting your partner know if you're feeling suffocated at any point. You'll want to, however, have a key signal, like two taps on her thigh, to indicate that she's getting carried away with any thrusting. This action is fun until you're choking on it! While a submissive position, remember that you're ultimately the one in charge.

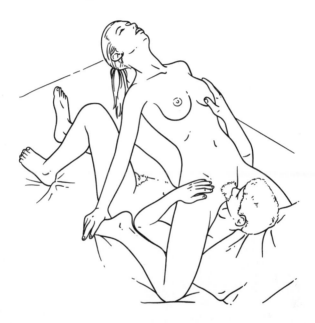

Variations:

- Have her hover over you instead of pulling a face plant.
- Change directions, meaning have her sit the other way in riding your face, especially if you want deeper tongue penetration of the anus. If you bend your legs, she can rest against your knees for support if desired.

- If she's really flexible, as the top, she can go back into what's known as the *bridge pose* in yoga, and take your penis into her mouth for an acrobatic version of 69!
- If she's tall enough, ask her to stand at the edge of the bed while sitting on your face.
- She can squat instead of kneel, but this probably won't be as comfortable and may pose the risk of her falling on you when she gets caught up in her climax.

Tips:
- She can prop herself up against a wall or a bed's headboard for more support and better balance.
- You can grip her buttocks to better control the thrusts.
- You can prop yourself up slightly with pillows for easier action.
- Don't try to "chase" her if she eases off your mouth or wants you to no longer focus on a particular hot spot. She's either trying to prolong the action or needs a bit of a "breather."

Sex Savvy

Face-sitting is not to be mistaken for a "pussy smother," a hardcore BDSM (bondage, discipline, sadomasochism) move which seeks to deprive the submissive lover of air. Get trained in domination and S&M if you are interested, as this is not to be practiced by amateurs!

| From Behind

Why couples love it: Anything rear entry is hot. Plus, you've got amazing access to smother yourself with her pussy.

Her: Get on all fours for your "tongue lashing." As you get more and more turned on, let your lover know by moving your hips, rhythmically, but gently "pushing back" to get more into the action (if he isn't into it or wants more control), he'll grab your hips in an effort to direct.

You: Approach your lover's genitals from behind. Point your tongue and thrust into her vagina, occasionally swirling the nerve-packed opening swiftly and firmly. If you're up for it, and she's into it, consider the same move with her anal opening.

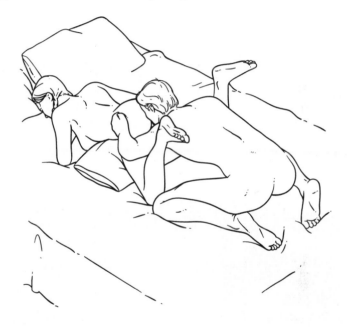

Variations:

- You can slide under her, face under genitals. Use your forearms to lift yourself against her body.
- She can provide a better angle by leaning down onto her forearms.

Tips:

- Take advantage of the fact that you may never have such great access to the perineum, digging your tongue, knuckle, fingertip, or a sex toy firmly into this hot spot, with a massaging motion, to unleash the sexual energy housed here.
- With the full exposure, given stimulation can be a bit intense, try a strong downward stroke.

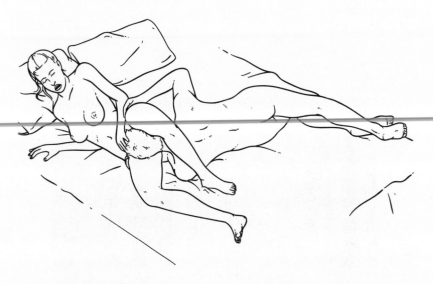

Sideways

Why couples love it: There's something about lounging around with a few nibblies.

Her: She lies down on her side. As she becomes more and more aroused, she should try rocking her body to and fro. Or, she can wrap one leg around your back to guide your rhythm, squeezing you toward her when she wants you buried in her even more.

You: Choose your angle, as some will allow for more shallow versus deeper action.

Tip:

- Experiment with just how far you want to part her legs, as this impacts how much you'll have to play with.

Variations:

- Both of you can be on your side.
- Approach giving from a perpendicular angle, with your partner lying in one direction across the bed and you the other. She can also lift her top leg for a more interesting variation and all access.

Sex Savvy

Note the arch of her back. This "hysterical arch," as it's known, is often featured as a major and typical part of female sexual response in porn flicks. But it is not natural. This arching actually cuts off the blood flow to her pelvic area, compromising her breathing and ultimately her sexual response. A woman who is sexually excited and comfortable will have a flat back, genitals slightly tilted towards her lover's mouth and not downward. This is made easier with a pillow or two under her neck and shoulders.

| Wrap Around

Why couples love it: This oral sex position allows for full body contact like no other.

Her: All she has to do is sit on a couch.

You: Sit behind her and wrap yourself around her. Now bend yourself around the one side of her body until your mouth reaches her clitoris. You'll ultimately end up on your side in performing oral, and will likely have to ask her to tuck her pelvis upward and pull her mons back for full clitoral exposure.

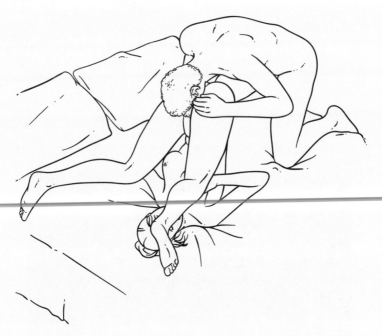

Plough Pose

Why couples love it: What can be more perfect than the meeting of zen and bliss?

Her: She's lying on her back, then, like the yoga pose, lifts her legs up straight in the air, her hands supporting her lower back, then swings her legs over her head. She may be able to touch her toes to the floor. Alternatively, she may be able to rest her knees close to her ears. **Note:** This is only for physically fit and flexible people (yoga experience preferred)!

You: You've got more direct access than you've ever imagined. You can kneel, sit, or stand and bend in making her moan. Go wild!

Tip: Check in with her to make sure she can breathe easily.

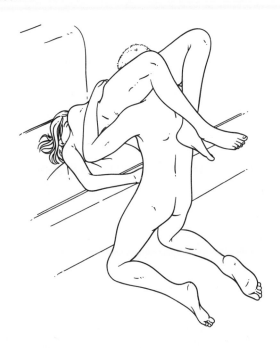

Bottoms Up!

Why couples love it: Airborne genitals feel freer.

Her: She's lying down with her legs over your shoulders.

You: Place your hands under her bum for added support.

Variations: Depending on your heights, you can try both sitting and standing while delivering.

Tips:

- Only attempt this if you're strong enough.
- If on your knees, be kind to yourself with a soft surface, e.g., rest on pillows.

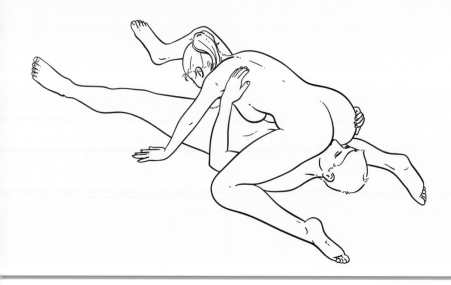

Soixante-Neuf "69"

Why couples love it: It holds the ooo-la-la of French sex appeal.

Receiver and Giver: You are both, so either lie on your sides or decide who is the top, facing the downward and the opposite direction. If there's a top, this person can guide the action.

Tip: Place a pillow under the bottom's head in cases where someone is on top.

Variations:

- Almost 69, which is where one partner simply isn't returning the favor.
- 68, where one partner lies down, face up, and the other lies the opposite way, also face up.

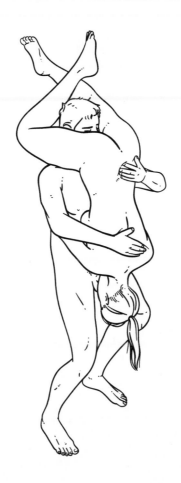

Standing 69

Meant for true athletes, standing 69 is more easily done moving from off of 69 on a high-standing bed. The "base" partner (all bets are that that's you) will need to exercise incredible strength in lifting the two of you off of the bed while keeping both of you interlocked in 69. Alternatively, you can approach this version of 69 with one partner assuming headstand while the other stands, supporting this partner's legs. The lover doing the headstand can then slowly be lifted so that mouths and groins meet. In either case, the partner who is upside down does best in gripping the thighs of the standing partner, while strongly squeezing his or her legs into the standing one's sides.

Sitting or Kneeling 69

Depending on how tall you and your lover are, you may want to try the kneeling 69, where the "base" partner kneels. Whether for greater comfort or stability, sitting on the side of a bed or chair is another variation. Finally, if you have or are a super flexible partner, have your lover bend over all the way as you sit on the floor for a more from behind angle. The upside-down partner can also spread his or her legs for variation. Note: If it's hard to have both of you pleasuring at the same time, have partners face the same direction for an advanced version of 68.

Finally, with her legs thrown over your shoulders, her arms wrapped back around your waist, you can stand with her pussy right in your face.

Sex Savvy

Don't beat yourself up if you're not bowled over by 69. While some find it absolutely delightful, others hold that it's not worth the trouble, as in too many distractions, too much going on, or too much to choreograph. Plus, the best part of oral sex can be losing yourself in your own pleasuring or in her!

| Erotic Furniture and Supports

Oral sex gives lovers the perfect excuse to consider their sex equipment. Pillows, props, bolsters, and other play gear can open lovers to a whole new realm of sexual pleasuring, especially in cases where movement is limited (e.g., pregnancy, or one person may be hurting). In planning ways you want to bend, suspend, prop up, move, or touch each other, consider the following in adding novelty and variety to your oral sex positions:

- **Sex Swing.** Hung over your closed door, this suspension's acrylic tubes are placed over the top of the door. You can then slip her legs into the loops, adjusting them on the thighs. The receiver then balances herself with arm handles while you do a little more than lick your lips.
- **Super Sex Sling.** For long-haul oral sex sessions, place this sling's thick pad behind the receiver's neck. You can then position her using an adjustable suspension strap, secured with Velcro cuffs.
- **Positioning Sex Strap.** For serious eat-me-out sex, the padded strap around her lower waist allows for a comfortable lift.
- **Sex Furniture.** Sold under brand names like Liberator Shapes and Love Pegasus, these soft, but firm padded platforms come in a variety of inclines, platforms, and shapes. Have fun exploring different sexual positions, including those that help to facilitate orgasm and lift the pelvis for better oral sex stimulation.

Sex Savvy

In restraining or suspending a partner, make sure that she experiences no muscle or joint stress. Blood flow and breathing shouldn't be restricted in any way. Arms and legs should not be left suspended for too long, or else the lack of blood flow will cause unpleasant sensations and numbing. The restraint should be safely secured, but not too tight. If that isn't the case, assist your lover in changing positions or adjust the restraint.

| Taking Your Show on the Road

You're ready to realize oral sex in the great outdoors, meaning anywhere but within the confines of your bedroom walls. So whether looking at your washing machine, balcony, or shower in a whole new way, or analyzing if oral sex feats involving a closet, car, plane, or train are well worth the risk, consider the following matters:

- **Mouth access**. Just how easy will it be for the lips and genitals to meet?
- **Depth**. How much of your lover's loins will make it into the mouth?
- **Angle**. Are you able to reach her major hot spots?
- **Space**. How much do you have to work with?
- **Comfort**. Will either of you be uncomfortable, especially if you plan to hold your position for a while?
- **Props**. Can the sexual scenario be made comfortable? Are any enhancements needed?
- **Fantasy component**. Other than shaking things up, and running the risk of getting into major trouble in some cases, what can make oral sex outside of the bedroom all that?

You should have plenty of opportunities to pull off many oral trysts all over the place, so don't fret too much about what you can pull off. Carpe diem! Just try it, realizing that getting frisky with some flirting and foreplay will better the pleasure to be added in any oral sex endeavor.

CHAPTER 4

Foreplay for Oral Sex

The adage "getting there is half the fun" has never been truer than when it comes to seduction. Few people can resist the allure of being lured by a lover, with attempts at the fine art of foreplay often more exciting than the eventual sex act of choice. In bringing the senses to life while stoking the fires of longing, foreplay is a dance between partners that seeks to drive them to the brink of sexual peaking. With anticipation lending itself to feverish amour, lovers up the ante of pleasures to be had orally in teasing each other to no end with various foreplay scenarios.

"My guy and I have an exclusively oral sex session at least once a week. We don't always have the energy for all out intercourse and oral sex is so exquisite in and of itself that we can't resist making it the main focus. The experience becomes that much more erotic when it's all we want to do, and has explosive results attained in no other way." }Jane

| Appetizer or Main Course?

Many lovers regard oral sex as a sexy longing to be satiated en route to "bigger and better" things. With intercourse largely seen as the main course of erotic exchanges between lovers, oral sex is often not given the full attention it deserves. Yet this sensual appetizer can very much be the main play instead of simply foreplay. In fact, making it so allows lovers to fully luxuriate in the experience, milking it for all that it is worth.

Instead of being consumed with what's to come, you can bask between her legs as a "cunnilinguist" or as the star of the show. No matter what your role, approaching oral sex as the main act takes pressure off, allowing you more opportunities to be intimate and bond, and more excuses to entice one another. Whether an act of foreplay or the "coreplay," oral action revs up your sexual response, and will often have you hungering for more.

Sex Savvy

Arrange for a date night that will involve no more than oral coreplay. Such pleasuring makes sex much less goal-oriented, taking the pressure off of lovers to get somewhere, and allowing them to simply enjoy the moment and the sex play at hand.

Getting Back to Basics: Kissing

In our eagerness to pucker up with one's privates, it can be easy to overlook the oral pleasures to be had with the original oral sex—kissing. Physical, emotional, and sexual: A great deal of information is exchanged when our lips meet. The kiss expresses a slew of feelings, like affection, passion, love, need, forgiveness, wanting, and missing. Men in particular use kissing as a way to seduce, and they're quite into puckering up— much more so than they're given credit for.

As a sexual act that is part of romantic and carnal passion in over 90 percent of the world's cultures, the kiss is a major mate-assessment tool and is rated as one of the most romantic acts a couple can partake in. Not surprisingly, kissing is directly proportional to a couple's relationship satisfaction. So whether you plan to make oral sex the foreplay or coreplay of a sexual session, remember that the original kiss is where you can perfect your technique before going for the genitals.

Sex Savvy

Kissing burns 26 calories per minute. With most people spending 20,160 minutes in a lifetime kissing, that's 524,160 calories burned!

Reasons Lovers Love Kissing

Kissing indicates to your lover that you're interested in being sexually intimate to some degree. It can also hint at what you have to offer in the oral department down there, with fan-yourself make-out sessions inspiring imaginations gone wild. That's part of what makes kissing so exciting, especially in situations where you're not sure just how far exchanges will erotically escalate. Caught up in the moment, you or your lover may be perfectly content playing tonsil hockey and find yourselves doing absolutely nothing more than locking lips. And this is perfectly fine since kissing serves to:

- Promote sexual access sooner or later, with males being particularly clever in using the kiss as a way to lasciviously lure romantic partners.
- Induce bonding and commitment.
- Show your genuine desire and love for another.
- Invite reconciliation, helping lovers to reunite after a fight.
- Trigger sexual desire with the exchange of testosterone.
- Spike dopamine in the brain, which is associated with romantic love. (The neurotransmitters released with a kiss are the same brain chemicals that go crazy when you sky dive or run a marathon!)
- Cause sexual excitement, which may increase levels of oxytocin in both men and women.

Research out of Lafayette College has found that kissing increases hormones in the brain, setting off a complex chemical process that makes the experience relaxing, exciting, and loving. While men have a heightened awareness of these feelings, women need extra ambiance, like dim lighting or romantic music, to reach the same state. Researchers aren't sure why this chemical reaction happens, but suspect that it's due to the swapping of hormones in the saliva.

Rolls Off the Tongue

"A great kiss is the ultimate aphrodisiac. If I'm dating someone who is an amazing kisser, I automatically assume that everything else is going to be amazing, including the oral. It's powerful and intoxicating, always leaving me wanting more." }Jaymes

Get Caught Up in Kissing

When it comes to oral endeavors, kissing is a way to mutually teach each other about the techniques you like. It's a way to learn about the rhythms, pressures, and stylistic approaches your lover might enjoy in more place than one. So set out to spend a date simply kissing and nothing else. Focus on the mouth as your prime pleasure center. Your mission: to discover exactly the way your lover wants to be kissed or to experiment with different kissing techniques and styles.

Take turns being the lead kisser. When it's her turn to be in charge, ask her to show you what she likes, or simply exhale "Do you like that?" as you come up to breathe from a smokin' make-out session. Pay attention, too, to her nonverbal compliments, what she's doing with her body to show you that she's into the experience. Erotically escalate the action by responding more enthusiastically with your own kissing. Lick and suck her tongue to plant ideas of what's to come. When taking breathers, lick your way down her treasure trail, stop short of her mons, smile and work your way back up. Repeat several times.

Sex Q & A

How can you get a lover to kiss you in a way that teaches them what you want done to your genitals? I love to give, but, naturally, I'm hoping she'll return the favor!

You can easily do this using a direct approach, simply saying, "I'd love it if you tried kissing me (or using your tongue this way) next time you go down on me." Most lovers appreciate, and even want, clear direction on what turns the other on. If you'd prefer to use a more indirect approach, however, exaggerate the style you desire in your own kissing, even hinting, "I'm so imagining you doing this somewhere else." Your lover will hopefully tune into the rhythm or technique you're trying to establish, realizing that this is what you want. Ask her to do the same if she has trouble telling you what she wants.

In giving ample attention to kissing, like with the other oral, be sure to take breathers, gazing into each other's eyes or sprinkling her face, neck, and shoulders with kisses. Keep the moment light with sweet nothings and appreciations. This can act as an incredible tease as to when exactly you may go south, if at all.

Lip Care for Better Loving

No matter what kind of kiss you're delivering, you want sexy lips. With a person's face often being the first thing that catches another's attention, mouth maintenance becomes critical in evoking positive reactions. Healthy, soft, luscious lips make you look appealing and attractive, a point made even more evident when you think about how having dry, chapped lips can impact one's look negatively. So alluring are the lips that the media can't get enough of featuring Hollywood stars who have luscious lips. Note: Men with perfectly pouty mouths can be quite delicious looking too. Looking kissable is irresistible, and this starts with proper lip care.

In making mouth maintenance a regular part of your self-care routine, drink plenty of water and eat a lot of vitamin-rich foods, like fruits and vegetables. Regularly apply lip balm or moisturizers year-round, with those containing SPF ideal for maximum sun protection when needed. Lip butter or an aloe lip treatment can also help with moisturizing, keeping your lips soft, soothed, hydrated, and protected. A lipscuff, like that made by the Body Shop, that removes dead skin, can further give you a conditioned feel.

Rolls Off the Tongue

"I think it's cute when a guy pays attention to lip care. It indicates that he thinks good presentation is important and wants to be able to do more than talk with those lips." } Hannah

| Oral Seductions

Beyond the art of kissing, in working your way to a lover's most titillating target zones, you want to build sensations and be a tease. Initiating oral action is your way to take sexiness to a whole new level. Any or a combination of the following seductive strategies are sure to make your partner putty in your hands for other oral attentions in no time.

Look Like You Want Sex

Beyond presentation, you want to look cool, calm, and collected, but ready to pounce when things rev up. This starts with giving a love interest longing glances, holding her gaze for a moment, and smiling invitingly. Touch places you'd like to be touched later, like your neck. Run your fingers through your hair or play with the buttons on your top. These are all, often unconscious, signals that you're attracted to another.

Sexy Q & A

How much foreplay is necessary for having good sex?

The amount of warm-up needed for good sex varies by lover and can differ from one situation to the next. A person who is stressed after a hard day at work may require more foreplay in getting in the mood for intimacy, while lovers who have been flirting all day via phone may be ready to get all over each other the moment they meet. In general, the amount of foreplay doesn't determine good sex so much as the quality of it. The brain is one of the biggest sex organs, so mental erotic engagement is more important than anything. Engaging the brain can take mere seconds or many minutes, and is very individual.

Let Your Lover Know You Want Sex

Establish a secret signal for those times you want only oral. This might be as simple as drawing an "O" on your lover's lower back to putting on an entire performance. In letting your lover know what you have in mind the next time you rendezvous, tape a flirtatious note to the peach in her lunch bag. Send her a sexy email, detailing all of the ways you plan to bring her to climax the next time you're on your knees. Whether subtle (e.g., licking your lips as though savoring them) or very direct (e.g., whispering "I hope you're not wearing any underwear right now") oral efforts are initiated when you get devilishly flirtatious and fresh.

Sex Savvy

Keeping things playful is key in maintaining sexual interest in the form of foreplay. Sex toy shops have numerous adult oral sex board games, adding tantalizing tasks to your adventures. They'll have you playing to win as never before, with games like the Oral Sex Board Game. The winner receives oral sex!

Take Charge

Exuding an attitude of playfulness, confidence, and hungering, let your needs be known. This *carpe diem* approach to stimulating desire can be as easy as putting on some music and slow dancing, drawing a sensual bath, playing a romantic movie, or popping in a sex tape capturing your last orgasmic oral endeavor. Remember, your approach sets the tone of the action to come as more romantic, spiritual, or lascivious.

Cover Her with Kisses

Whether spread out on your bed or lying across your dining room table, cover your partner's body with kisses, intentionally avoiding the areas aching for the most attention. Take your time attending to hot spots everywhere else but the most volcanic ones, teasing these areas with your tongue, massaging them with your lips, or sucking on them to the point you almost leave a hickey.

Sex Savvy

Get a little crazy with your kissing, trying moves beyond the traditional kiss. This might include tugging your lover's bottom lip with your teeth. Or sucking on her tongue when it's in your mouth. Or tickling the roof of her mouth with your tongue. With every move, consider how it could be incorporated into your oral efforts.

Use Your Hands

Warm up your partner's genitals with a nice erotic massage. Bring your lover's erogenous zones to life with some finger action, starting gently at first and slowly building the pace while gradually applying more pressure. Incorporate some of your favorite lubricant, making things wet in a way that's sexually suggestive.

Seduce with Sound

Stimulate your partner's auriculogenital reflex (ear stimulation response) by breathing heavily into her ear. Or practice some sultry sex talk, like "I have to have you," getting as graphic or as dirty as you think your lover can handle.

Practice Fresh Breath

It's hard to maintain cool breath when gum isn't the best idea pre-oral. You can, however, whip out a fresh breath spritz like Binaca. Tasting like peppermint, spearmint, or cinnamon only makes your mouth all the more inviting for all over the body.

Slip in a Naughty Movie

Sometimes you need help planting the seed or launching sexual excitement. A steamy flick, X-rated or not, can do just the trick in getting a lover's mind on more important matters.

Rolls Off the Tongue

"I feel like more of a sex goddess when I have oral sex in the shower. In being totally naked and wet, I feel wilder, more in tune with my original form. The water running in and out of my mouth as we kiss or when I give makes me feel even more carried away, and I can easily get carried away with these fantasies of where we're becoming one with nature." —Sara

| Lathering Up: Bath and Shower Play

Sometimes all the seduction you need for oral is a little bit of water play. Some lovers need to wash up before oral, mentally cleansing themselves more than anything. Others like the excuse of getting fresh while freshening up. Even if a shower or bath isn't necessary, it's hard to resist getting naked and running your hands all over a lover's slick body. Getting glimpses of your lover's private parts amidst the soap suds of a bubble bath can have you all the more eager for her warm wetness. Lovers can hardly resist lathering up, hands gliding over the other's sex as they bathe or shower together. It's only natural for the mouth to follow . . . .

Adding to the appeal of water play is that it gives the perfect excuse to try positions not usually done in bed during oral pursuits, like standing. The warm water also has a relaxing, but invigorating effect, encouraging lovers to release the day's tensions and let loose in a most uninhibited way. Finally, the wetness may allow you to bypass the need for lube while still keeping things slick.

| Don't Forget the Ambiance!

It should go without asking, but often because of that, it can be overlooked: Are you in a seductive environment? A little can do a lot when it comes to the overall experience and her receptivity to your oral efforts. Any well thought out sexual rendezvous can turn you into quite the entertainer if your location is lusty.

There are tons of things you can do to make your place visually and sexually stimulating. Start by tearing down your collage of buxom Carmen Electra girlie posters—a guaranteed turn-off for her. You should also hide pictures of exes, old sports heroes, and pop stars, and give your place a complete décor makeover in general.

Strive to give your pad (especially your room) a good cleaning, changing your sheets and adjusting the lights low to really set the mood. Remember, shadows can be so alluring, especially since she may not be down with you going down on her with the lights on—at least not initially.

Finally, consider your choice of music as an environmental aphrodisiac. The two of you can get drunk on music if you're in the right mood and looking for the perfect, lust-filled atmosphere, whether it's heavy metal for something hardcore or jazz for a more sensual seduction.

Rolls Off the Tongue

"When it comes to any kind of sex, for me, it's daylight or lights definitely ON!! But I don't think I would feel this way in a new relationship. I think it would take a while with someone new to be comfortable enough to have the lights on. But as the relationship ages, I think people become more comfortable with themselves around their lover." } Samantha

| Role-Playing

When it comes to your erotic imagination, anything can happen—and almost anything can be acted out. Fantasies and sexual storylines can stir one's libido, bolster sexual excitement, and add new life to oral sexplorations. In a relationship defined by trust, good communication, openness, and a sense of adventure, sharing your phantasms for role-play during foreplay can be an erotically intense bonding experience. While it can be a bit intimidating and embarrassing to share some of our deepest curiosities, longings, and desires, dishing out sexual imaginings for live, passion-filled performances can make for some of the most memorable moments. As you ponder which storylines to share (and not), and which scenarios have the potential for bedroom theater, consider, too, the following orally themed sexual fantasies in launching your riveting role-play efforts.

- **Virgin Sex**. Your lover has never given oral sex before and is most eager to be mentored. Be a good teacher and give this newbie plenty of erotic instruction on how to go down on you. Or as the "virgin" giver, be sure to ask for more detailed directions, playing up what you don't know and exaggerating your reactions as to what it's like to lick, taste, and be the perfect pleaser.

- **Stranger Sex.** Plan to meet at a bar, only pretend that you don't know each other. If you're the one hitting on the other, simply say "hello," offer to buy this eye candy of yours a drink, make small talk, then ask if she wants to get out of there for a little fun. Don't say a word as you steal off to a secluded location. Your sole focus and concern: giving or receiving the best "anonymous" oral ever.

- **Cop and Careless Driver.** You've just been pulled over for reckless driving. You know you're guilty, but can't afford the ticket and want to avoid jail time. How are you going to get yourself out of the situation? It may simply require offering the nice looking lady officer some serious oral sex in the back seat of your car.

- **Psychotherapist and Client.** Normally, you would never think to act inappropriately in taking advantage of a distraught client, but this case is classic Freudian and you have a few ideas on how to best treat this person's arrested development when it comes to oral fixations.

- **Bad Girl/Boy Scenario.** You've been a bad boy. The best form of "punishment": going down on her. Maybe that will teach you to be "bad" again.

- **Dracula Sex.** While your victim's neck is irresistible, there's an erogenous zone you'd rather suck and lick and satiate. In making sure that your victim doesn't get away while being "tortured," be sure to tie her up with restraints, like a scarf or handcuffs. Enhance oral efforts by focusing your lover's attention with a blindfold. Available in soft black microfiber, pleather, leather, silk, and satin, among a host of other fabrics, this tool will force your partner to tune into the sensations, getting more out of the experience.

"I would never want to hook up with another woman, but the fantasy I have of a dominatrix succumbing to me by going down on me is one of my favorites." } Kendra

Oral Sex Phantasms

Research on oral sex regularly confirms that giving or receiving oral sex is one of most common fantasies. People may fantasize about oral sex while masturbating or while having sex with their partner. Ask anybody willing to share, and they'll often confess that their sexual fantasies have included some type of oral ongoings, including having a same sex partner go down on them, anonymous oral sex, oral sex orgies, and 69.

"Oral sex orgy-style fantasies are some of the hottest I have. Naked, oiled up people all feasting on each other's loins and taking turns on each other. . . . it's so taboo and uncommon and racy in being considered so wrong. And it *so* gets me off!" } Magda

On Location

Bold lovers will sometimes take their show on the road, engaging in oral sex in secluded locations or in very public places where action is still quite discreet. In brainstorming all of the places where you might be able to get away with some oral action, consider that getting busted could land you in some legal trouble in such exhibitionism being illegal. Still, with the risk of getting caught a huge part of the erotic thrill, lovers have bragged about where they've been willing to engage in oral, with the following some of the most popular:

- In your backyard
- In a car
- In a movie theater
- At the beach
- At the car wash
- At work
- In an elevator

Rolls Off the Tongue

"My ex-girlfriend had a wild side when it came to oral and was big on seeing what she could get away with when we'd go for picnics, whether while hiking, at the park, on the beach. . . . Having a blanket always helped, especially in allowing me to more boldly return the favor." }

Loren

CHAPTER 5

Techniques for Oral Sex Aficionados

When it comes to erotic inspiration, new techniques are seen as a way to avoid boredom, revive passion, and make for completely different experiences. Changing up the tried and true can be an enjoyable conquest, with variety offering novel experiences that keep lovers engaged, turned on to oral, and feeling united. For lovers new to orally pleasuring each other, employing different tactics during their trial-and-error period helps them to discover what the other is into. No matter what the situation, techniques for oral sex add spice for never-before-known sensations, upping one's oral aptitude for impressing any lover.

Rolls Off the Tongue

"My girlfriend and I admittedly try some of those oral sex tips you read about in magazines like *Cosmo*. Sometimes they do nothing for us. Other times, it's like *wow*! Give me more of that!" }Paul

| Warming Up the Vulva

In going down on a woman, you'll want to warm her up a bit first. While it's tempting to go for the gold—her clitoris—the entire vulva needs some attending to first. But before you even get to that, tease her a bit with loving kisses on her belly or by making long, gentle strokes with your tongue from her knees to her pubes. Use just the smoother underside of your tongue across the inside of her thighs. Repeat several times.

As you start to home in on her vulva, press the mons pubis in a downward direction to indirectly awaken the area before covering the vulva with all of your mouth. You can also give it a good massage, rubbing it easily at first, and then with more pressure, in a clockwise rotation.

Send shivers down her spine by dragging your fingers up and down her inner thighs, selectively planting kisses to the area around her groin, acting as a tease for what's to come. In getting her wetter and warmer, start by giving the vulval area long licks, as though thoroughly enjoying an ice cream cone. Starting at the base of her vaginal entrance, work your way up to the top of the clitoral hood, for a light "drive by" before working your way back down on the other side. For different sensations, use little cat-like licks instead of a bigger sweeping motion. Have a finger trail your action for the hard versus soft contrast of a tongue versus digit. Save the clitoral hood for last.

| Oral Sex Basics

When it comes to her pleasuring, a number of techniques can be used to awaken, accelerate, and amplify arousal in stimulating another's genitals with the mouth. Major moves include licking, lapping, flicking, slurping, circling, tickling, sucking, kissing, pressing, and nibbling a particular hot spot or her whole vulva. The pace can be anywhere from fast to slow, with pressure anywhere from hard to soft. Patterns of movements across erogenous zones can be side to side, up-down, diagonal, or circles. Pick up any popular magazine and you'll likely be dared to skillfully try drawing the alphabet or figure eights with the tip of your tongue in getting the blood down there flowing even more.

The key in figuring out what your gal enjoys is to add a little variety from one sex session to the next. Changing up the technique also works in prolonging sexual intimacy. In other words, if you don't want her to come right away or if you want this sexual moment to last, avoid too much attention on her clitoris and switch things up. For example, you can experiment with different parts of the mouth to create different sensations, like repeatedly rubbing the really soft inside of the lips across an erogenous zone for an exquisite eroticism. Various parts of the tongue, namely the top, sides, tip, and under part, can make for an entirely different experience as well, especially because you can make it soft, pointed, or firm.

No matter what you choose to do, start out slowly, building up the rhythm. Keep in mind that maintaining consistency when it comes to pressure and pace, including kicking it up a notch or two, is what brings a lover to orgasm. You want to take your time getting to one that works for her in warming her up first. You'll throw her for a loop, disrupting her concentration and ability to get into the sensations if you dive right in or hastily change from one technique to the next. Making, then breaking, contact from time to time can, though, help to build sexual tension when done skillfully.

More than anything, as you work to make her putty in your hands, maintain your enthusiasm. Being into it, even if you're not, can be what means more to her than anything else going on. If your enthusiasm level is related to your confidence level when it comes to giving, then don't let any doubts hold you back. Once again, fake it until you can make it happen for real. You're not hurting anybody in acting like you know what you're doing. You're only making the experience better for her in taking your time, keeping your cool, and feeling good about yourself and what's going on.

| Attending to the Clitoris

As long as she's aroused, her clitoris should be coming to life. But instead of zeroing in on it, flirt with this hot spot a bit, gently massaging it with a wet finger. Add more pressure to these light touches before having your tongue make contact, keeping it relaxed at first. If you'd rather not use your finger, you can hover over her clitoris and glide your lips over it just to tease, then pull back and repeat several times. In any case, slowly increase the rhythm and pressure of your movements, bringing it completely to life before attempting any of the following:

- Press your flattened tongue over her clitoris hard and wiggle it to and fro while shaking your head "no," slowly and tenderly at first.
- Use firm, brisk horizontal or vertical licks across the clitoris.
- Swirl your tongue around the clitoris several times, then suck.
- Use a "v" motion/"reverse v" around the clitoris.
- Suck on the clitoris as you flick your tongue's tip across it or push up against it, or circle. If she can handle it, take her clit between your teeth.
- Make small, purposeful circles on either side of the hood with your tongue.
- Take her clitoris into your mouth and just suck, experimenting with different suction pressures in seeing what she likes, or rather what she can handle.
- Caress her clitoris, making love to it in much the same way you do her tongue in French kissing her.
- Harden your tongue into a point and dart it back and forth across the clit. As she gets more excited, "bang" it up against the clit rhythmically.
- Use the underside of your tongue over her clitoral hood.
- If she can handle it, pull back her clitoral hood gently and, using an upward motion, stroke the tip of her clit with your tongue. Note: This may make her hypersensitive. Alternatively, you can press the heel of your hand into the top of her mons pubis to naturally retract the hood for more direct action.

If at any point you want to strategize your next move or need a breather, work your way to the vaginal opening, point your tongue and put it in and out of the vaginal opening for some "tongue fucking." Occasionally, swirl your tongue around the vulva or come up to blow hot air from your gut or cool air on her groin (lower abs, inner thighs, and outer genitals).

| Making Use of Your Hands

Sometimes, your tongue may be all she needs—all the stimulation that she can handle. Other times, you'll both want your hands to get in on the act, stimulating other hot spots and expanding climactic sensations throughout the body. So try:

- Sliding both hands under her bum, gripping her cheeks firmly as you make long, luscious laps over her clit.
- Use only one hand to grip her bum, making use of your fingers on the other (as we'll get to in a second).
- Shift a hand supporting her bum so that you can massage her perineum with your thumb. Have her press her thighs together, in varying the sensation, as you focus on her mons and clitoral hood.
- Depending on your position, massage her butt cheeks, perhaps in rhythm with your tongue movements. Have them run down the back of her thighs.
- Reach up and cup and massage her breasts, running your hands down her sides when your arms feel tired.
- Slip a vibrator into her vaginal entrance (apply lube first, if necessary), pressing it into the area about two inches up from the vaginal opening (her G-spot area). You can also use the vibe in a gentle thrusting motion, or have it circle her opening, which is lined with nerve endings. Finally, don't forget that the vibe can be used on

her clit, especially if you're wanting a bit of a break, but not wanting to interrupt stimulation of this prime hot spot.

- Press your thumb against her anal opening, massaging it with the tip.

| Finger Play

Multitasking has never been so sexy. As you go down on her, have your fingers playing with her as well, employing erotic techniques like the following:

- Insert one of your first two fingers partway into her vaginal opening. Firmly, and as though luxuriously, have it circle her vaginal entrance. As she starts to warm up to this action, place another finger in the entrance area, and slowly work your way up the front wall of her vaginal canal. You're feeling for a rough, raised area—her G-spot. Once you've found this area, firmly massage it in a clockwise or counterclockwise motion. Alternatively, you can rub it from side to side or up and down, checking in with her as to what she likes.
- Focusing on her G-spot, use a "come hither" motion with a finger or two in stroking it, as this is the most effective way to awaken it for many women.
- Anytime you go farther south to orally stimulate the vaginal opening, her perineum, or anus, keep a thumb tip against her clitoral hood. You can lightly massage it or have it rhythmically tap up against her clitoral area.
- Press down on her pubic mound as you work your tongue across her clit diagonally.
- Rock your finger tip back and forth across the clitoris, applying pressure directly on or from the side (closer to the base).

- If she can handle it—and likes it—try smacking up against her clit with the base of your palm or slapping it with your fingers.
- Gently take her clit between your thumb and forefinger and rub it as though you were rolling a little ball of paper. Or squeeze it intermittently, in rhythm with your tongue movements.
- Rock the heel of your hand across her clitoris or mons pubis.
- Rub, tug, or stroke her vaginal lips.

If you don't want her to cum sooner than later—and are feeling like teasing her a bit—pull back on direct clitoral (and/or G-spot) action. Slow down or halt tongue movements altogether. Pull away from her clit for a couple of seconds, then reapply pressure. Repeat until both of you can hardly contain yourselves in wanting more!

No matter your movements or mindblowing multitasking, be sure to check in with her regularly, asking things like, "Is this too intense?" "Does this hurt?" "Do you want more pressure here?" "Do you like that?" "Want more of that?" Also, don't underestimate the power of compliments. Letting her know how sexy, beautiful, and amazing she is at that very moment is going to not only make her feel that much better about the situation, but it will also leave her wanting more!

Sex Savvy

If your gal has a piercing, be careful with your teeth. If possible, flip the jewelry out of the way. Otherwise, consider how the piercing can add to the stimulation factor.

Tongue Kung Fu

Tongue Kung Fu is an ancient Chinese approach to skillfully and consciously giving or receiving oral sex. It's where you skillfully combine the use of your tongue, teeth, lips, and purpose in providing pleasure to bolster feelings of connectedness and passion. The following are some of the major techniques pursued:

- **Tongue Diving.** Using the full length and strength of your tongue, you directly "dive" into your lover's groin. Such an act is seen in this ancient Chinese art as expressing your love, since the tongue is seen as an extension of the heart.
- **Tongue Flutters.** Rapidly flutter your tongue back and forth across your lover's hot spots, as though this muscle is a vibrator.
- **Tongue Scooping.** Form your tongue in a spoon shape to use in a "come hither" motion on a hot spot, like her perineum.

In finding her pleasure, consider that some women really enjoy quick strokes across the clit. Others may prefer that their inner lips be firmly tugged so as to indirectly work that hot spot. Such indirect stimulation is especially important to make note of for those times her clitoris hits sensory overload and your direct touch has become a bit too much to bear. If she can handle it, change things up, making sure all of her little genital gems are played with, by stroking, rubbing, tickling, sucking, nibbling, or tugging at them.

Sex Savvy

Unless your lover is into it, avoid giving hickeys or using your teeth, especially to the point of leaving bite marks. Ask if your lover finds either of these forms of stimulation a turn-on before leaving her black and blue!

Oral Sex Made Easier

No matter what your game plan, events may take an unexpected turn. Issues may come up that have the potential to throw off your game. Be open to anything, ready for anything. In gauging if things are going well, tune into your lover's sounds and bodily reactions. Ask, if it's not obvious whether or not she is thoroughly enjoying herself. Finally, don't be afraid to incorporate maneuvers and sex tips that come to you on the spot, like licking in rhythm to music that's playing, or humming to become your own vibrating sex toy, or twisting your tongue in ways your genes allow. Who knows what could end up feeling good? Approach your oral sex efforts as the sky is the limit.

Rolls off the Tongue

"I've found that what works for one lover might not for the next. Instead of being insulted, I've tried to be flexible and it's worked out best for both of us. It also helps to keep that in mind when I'm giving a lover feedback. They're not as likely to be insulted, but receptive to what works for me."

}Alex

Homework Suggestion

We just went over a bunch of different techniques, so it's natural that your head may be spinning. Your mouth may be salivating. If you're the sort who prefers a direct road map in getting places instead of venturing out on your own, this guide seeks not to disappoint. While each woman is sure to have her own preferences for what to do and how to do it, this step-by-step guide is usually a sure fire way to please her:

1. While getting her warmed up with some foreplay will certainly help your efforts, if you're looking to get right to the treats, begin with kissing her inner thighs slowly and sensually. Work your way toward

her clitoris, using your tongue as you go. Flood her vaginal area with tons of wet French kisses, devouring her as though insatiable.

2. Lick her inner and outer lips, slowly tracing them with the tip of your tongue. Retrace them again and again, only using a teasing, massaging motion with your tongue. Work your way up to her clitoral hood, giving it a couple sweeps of the tongue before making your way further south again.

3. Once you've teased her to no end, start tonguing her clitoris with a quick darting and/or thrusting movement. If this is a bit too much for her, press your lips around her clitoris and suck or lick it intensely. If she needs more indirect stimulation, do the same to her inner lips instead, which will trigger a reaction from the clitoral hood.

4. Every now and then, ease off from such intense stimulation, and focus on other parts of her genital region or cover her stomach with kisses, especially if she's pleading for a slight break. Let her know how incredibly hot and beautiful she is—how much you love going down on her. Tell her how good she tastes and how sexy her hot pussy is.

5. Gradually, work your way back to her clitoris and slowly flick your tongue horizontally across it, gradually gaining speed. You can also move your tongue upward from the vaginal opening to the clitoris and then across the clitoris. Vary your pressure and intensity by first keeping your tongue soft and gently caressing it, then tightening it into somewhat of a point and rhythmically licking it. Feel free to use wide, sweeping strokes or to completely zero in on it, all the while checking in with her and watching her facial expressions and bodily reactions to ascertain what feels good.

6. Once you've homed in on her hottest spot, use a steady rhythm to work her to climax. The insertion of one or two, preferably lubricated or licked, fingers into the vagina or anus while you're doing

this will provide an even greater stimulation for your lady, often sending her over the edge.

Sexy Q & A

My partner is pregnant and her sex drive is out of control! I'm loving it, but am needing to go down a lot more on her in keeping up. I am finding myself wondering if going down on a pregnant woman requires a different approach at all.

A number of pregnant women find that sexual intimacy during pregnancy is some of the best because their nether regions are more engorged with blood, and therefore more sensitive. Many have their first experiences with orgasm or multiple orgasms during this time, with oral sex being one way couples discover what her sexual response has to offer her. Oral sex on your gal may not need to change at all, or it may require less stimulation on your part. Forms of stimulation that were ineffective before may do wonders now. Likewise, former faves of hers may not be worth revisiting until after she has delivered. More than anything, you need to communicate with her about what feels good, what she wants, what she can handle, and what you can do to make oral some of the most amazing and memorable action of this time in her life.

| Is She Enjoying Herself?

It can be hard to tell if she's responding well to your efforts—that is, if she isn't panting, having trouble speaking, or screaming her head off. In noting if you're headed in the right direction, see if she's:

- Flaring her nostrils
- Squeezing her eyes
- Experiencing a sex flush

- Looking possessed
- Seemingly weak, her body soft from the pleasure
- Producing more vaginal fluid
- Pressing or grinding into your mouth
- Flexing rhythmically
- Sweating

Other good indicators that she's a little more than sexually aroused include a pounding heart, grabbing at your head or hair, deeper breathing, or holding in more tightly in one way or another.

Sexy Q&A

What are some moves to incorporate during rimming?

In eating her out during analingus, you may want to suck or circle the area of the anal opening. You can also dip your tongue into the opening. At the end of the day, you can basically use a lot of the same mouth, lip, and tongue moves that you would during other types of oral stimulation, depending on your lover's preferences. You may, though, have to spend more time stroking your partner's clitoris in keeping your lover relaxed, as the vulnerability factor of rimming can make her more anxious during this type of oral action.

| Afterplay

You're basking in the glow of some out of this world oral sex, but don't let things end there! Just as with other types of sex, afterplay is an important way to top off a satisfying experience, helping the feelings and sensations last. So instead of falling asleep or making for the door, kiss and hold each other afterward. Take a bath or shower together while on your sex high. Talk about how nice that was, especially if she's trying to get over issues with oral sex. Allow yourselves the chance to recharge, because, like delicious dessert, you never know when you just have the room to have a little bit more.

Rolls Off the Tongue

"Coming down from oral sex is one of the most magical parts of it. It's like you're in your own world and you have all of these feel-good chemicals coursing through your body. Lingering helps them to stay a little longer." }Charlotte

It's Playtime! Sensual Enhancements

What's in your sexual treasure chest? After reading this chapter, you may just have to add to it, as the occasional investment in erotic enhancements can do wonders for your sex life. Treating yourselves to practically anything of the "for adults only" assortment can introduce new sensations, variety, and lust-filled experiences when it comes to your oral efforts. With the sexual and sensual accoutrements numbering into the thousands, sorting through what's best for your passionate pleasuring can feel overwhelming. Here, we seek to make your next online or in-store sexy shopping experience all the easier and sex savvier, highlighting the most tempting goodies when it comes to oral sex

| Lubricants for Luscious Loving

You want it even wetter. Even though she has her own arsenal for keeping it wet, she's with you on that one. But which lube to use is a common question from lovers since there are so many types of lubricants on the market. Making matters even more confusing is knowing which ones are best for oral sex. Ample amounts of lube can enhance your oral experiences, so, without further ado, here are your choices.

Flavored Lubricants

Found at drugstores, adult shops (both online and physical), and other retail stores with sexual health products, flavored lubes were originally developed to help mask the smell and taste of condoms, primarily during oral sex. Latex safe, they can be used with sex toys as well. Depending on your preferred brand and flavor, the scent and taste can enliven the senses, making oral sex a more appetizing event. Oral sex becomes a completely different delectable dining experience when made more scrumptious with sensual "seasonings" of sorts, like mojito peppermint, pomegranate vanilla, and chocolate orange blends offered by sex toy companies like Babeland.

Flavored lubes do, however, have their drawbacks, in that they can:

- Dry quickly (though with saliva or water, they can become slick again).
- Stain sheets or be hard to wash if they're a certain color.
- Be too sticky for other forms of sex, like self-pleasuring.
- Irritate the skin of women who are sensitive to products used in the vaginal area.
- Invite a yeast infection, depending on the ingredients, namely glycerin. (So be sure to look for a water-based formula that is glycerin- and paraben-free.)

Be sure to test the products before use, testing for allergies by dabbing a spot on an area of your inner arm and hers for a potential reaction. If you're good to go, have a ball trying different ones to see which ones you and your partner like best. Brands like ID Flavored Lube offer a Sampler 10-Pack. Look for samples and variety packs from your favorite brands.

Sex Savvy

Lacking oral secretions? A moisturizing spray called Biotene is available for patients who don't produce saliva due to illness, medical treatment, age, and other such factors. Talk to your doctor about potential issues you're having with dry mouth, and if such a product is right for you.

Other Lubricant Options

If flavored lube isn't your thing, look into these varieties:

- **Water-based lubricants.** Though they tend to dry faster than other types of lubes, water-based lubricants tend to be the most user-friendly, i.e., nonirritating, and easy to clean off, overall.
- **Silicone lubes.** While these can be used, ingesting too much can lead to upset stomach. If you want to do silicone, make sure it's a high-quality one, as in free of cyclopentasiloxane, which can sometimes taste a bit like petroleum.
- **Oil-based lubricants.** These should not be used if you're practicing safer sex since these can compromise the latex. And even if you're not using a condom or dental dam (a rectangular sheet of, typically, latex, placed over the vulva or anal opening) applying an oil-based lube for oral action can be gross. Use at your own risk.
- **Warming lubricants.** Available in flavors like hot buttered rum and blueberry, these lubes heat up when you rub them onto your lover's body. Blow on the area to heat things up even more. Just be sure to test an area of your partner's skin first, as some people do not like the sensations these lubes provide.

Sexy Q & A

Is it okay to use Altoids in going down on a woman?

Whether using the breath mints or the Linger Internal Vaginal Flavoring both known as Altoids, users should be wary about using such products during cunnilingus. Both are just regular mints, meaning they're made out of sugar. While Linger promises to influence a woman's "internal feminine flavoring," slipping it into her vagina for oral sex is supposed to be for novelty use only. Putting sugar directly into the vagina can affect its natural pH balance, resulting in a yeast infection.

Edible Aphrodisiacs

After a more savory seductive experience? Aphrodisiacs are any food, drink, drug, scent, or item believed to attract, invite sexual desire, or increase your level of sexual excitement. So it can basically be anything you and your gal find stimulating, giving you a great deal of power over what edibles to introduce to oral efforts. Plus, experimenting with different edibles only adds to the adventure, helping lovers to bond more than anything.

In deciding on the aphrodisiac of your choice, you may want to consider some of the most popular of all time for upping your oral efforts:

- **Champagne.** Drizzle some sparkling wine on your partner's abdomen, and have fun chasing the streams of bubbly—in their many directions—with the tip of your tongue.
- **Fruit.** Between their suggestive shapes, textures, and juices, you can have a field day with fruits in suggesting where you want to take the action or making things a wee bit tastier. Rub sticky juices from fruit like papaya, peach, orange, and mango on your lover's groin—only to lick it all off.
- **Chocolate.** Acclaimed throughout the ages for its supposed sexual effects, this sweet makes lovers happier thanks to its key ingredients: caffeine, anandamide and phenylethylamine (PEA) (a natural antidepressant), and theobromine, which boosts endorphin production for a body high. Heat edible dark, white, and milk chocolates, available as novelty body paints, and apply all over your lover's body as tasty foreplay before the coreplay. Alternatively, you can melt chocolate body fondue and paint it all over her for sweet seduction. Smear body icing or pour chocolate syrup down your lover's treasure trail for an even tastier treat. In any case, consider going for dark chocolate, since it's known to be a vasodilator, increasing blood flow throughout the body, including the genitals.

| Accessories for Oral Pleasuring

In addition to edibles, there are a whole host of sex toys designed specifically for oral pleasuring or suggested for use in addition to your lips and tongue. Have a blast adding to the sensations or taking them to an entirely new level with some of the following:

Tongue vibe. Slip this vibrating tongue ring onto your tongue for tingly action. Available in glow-in-the-dark, this vibe has a powerful two-speed setting. Lingo is a waterproof, disposable version of the tongue vibrator, held in place with a stretchy band. The

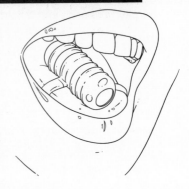

long-lasting motor of either brand is ideal for if and when your tongue ever gets tired.

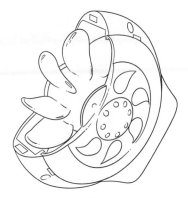

Sqweel. Double the oral action. Packed with ten soft, velvety tongues, this rotating wheel flicks across her hot spots. This battery-powered toy doesn't vibrate, but the wheel rotates to one of three speed options.

Sex Savvy

Never slip a dildo or vibrator into her vagina after you have used it for anal penetration, as this can invite infection. Be sure to thoroughly wash the toy with warm soap and water first or change condoms, if you're using such.

G-spot vibrator. Made specifically to hit this prime erogenous zone, various vibes are designed with a curved shaped to easily reach her G-spot. Experiment with the various speeds in seeing just how responsive her G-spot can be.

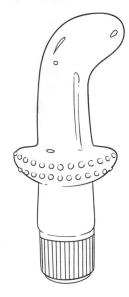

Dildo. Fulfill a third-party fantasy by slipping this toy into her nether crevices for full penetration, without the vibration, during oral sex.

Butt plug. Available in different sizes and shapes (ribbed, smooth, or bumpy), slowly insert this toy into the anus for more fullness during tongue action. Alternatively, you can thrust the butt plug in and out of her as you tease the clitoris. Note: Make sure your butt plug has a flared base so that it doesn't accidentally slip inside. Don't be surprised, too, if it shoots out as she reaches climax.

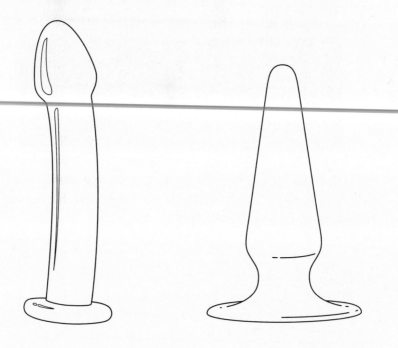

Anal beads. To intensify her orgasm, have anal beads in place, ready to stimulate the nerve endings of her anus, while giving her a nice nether massage. These typically five plastic or latex beads are strung together on a nylon or cotton cord. You want to insert each into her rectum, using lots of lube, one at a time while stimulating her clit. As she starts to approach climax, leisurely, gently, coax them out, by pulling at the ring at the end, with sweet and subtle tease-me tugging motions. For a more coordinated orgasm effort, postpone pulling them all the way out until your partner nears climax and let the last one slip out as she peaks.

> ## Sex Savvy
>
> Keep anal beads clean by putting a condom over them and knotting the end of the condom. You can also stick with nylon strings and latex beads since these are best when it comes to cleanliness and disinfecting. Oh, and it practically goes without saying, but never substitute any random objects, like ping pong balls, when it comes to this kind of sex play.

Climax Beads. More popularly known as Ben Wa balls, vaginal balls can be used much like anal beads in stimulating her vaginal canal. Like anal beads, these are available in a variety of sizes. Slowly pull these out of her as she hits heaven, encouraging her to flex her pelvic floor muscles as each ball slips out of her.

Rolls Off the Tongue

"We use sex toys on occasion for variety, especially for those times when you're in the mood, but don't want to do all of the work. The toys are a good excuse for those times we want to pleasure, but are feeling a bit lazy. Nobody is insulted. Both of us are happy." } Bobby

Restraints

We're eroticized by power, and bringing real world intensities into the bedroom can take oral sex in a whole new direction in tying her to the bed posts, donning a blindfold for added effect. But before experimenting with bondage and discipline, review the following checklist:

- Do you have a "safe" word? This is a word couples have agreed upon to stop all action, e.g., "apple" or "red." Though a safe word is a requirement of bondage and domination and sadomasochistic sex play, it's not such a bad idea to have one for those times you want to put a halt to the action.
- Have you negotiated the details of what you will and won't do? Lovers need to be clear about each other's needs. Likewise, they need to honor and respect their own and the other's limits.
- Is your restraint safe? You don't want to use just anything, as many binds can cause harm and injury. You want the restraints in place to be more for psychological effect than anything. Stick with wrist restraints and cuffs from reputable sex toy shops that are meant specifically for safe bondage play. Then make sure that your lover is comfortable and that blood is flowing into the hands before embarking upon your B&D adventures.

Sexy Q & A

My girlfriend is feeling a little nervous about supposedly "desensitizing" her private pleasure zone with too much vibration and artificial stimulus during oral sex. Can that really happen?

Women who use a vibrator report a more voracious sexual appetite, which tends to rise with increased use of their little love machines. These women claim that vibrator use actually enhances their overall sexual experiences, reassuring researchers that their vibrators were not necessary for orgasm, merely a means to stoke the flames. While the clitoris can feel overstimulated by a vibe at times, using one of these toys isn't going to ruin the nerve endings in this area.

Other Goodies

Massage mitt. Found at spas, sex toy shops, or your local drugstore, these love gloves of sorts come in different textures, like fur and stubs, for true magic hands.

Sex furniture. Sold under name brands like Liberator Shapes and Love Pegasus, padded platforms promise better sex, including oral sex. These soft props lift lovers for easier stimulation, allowing for better angles. Sliding one under your lover's bum, for example, can make for hotter analingus when her knees are pulled into the chest. In having her get on all fours, placing a prop under her lower abdominals can make for easier access to her private parts. You may just find that using these padded cushions makes for more orgasmic experiences.

Sport sheet. Going to bed never sounded so good with these bondage sheets. Used as regular bed sheets, they typically come with four Velcro restraints, one at each corner, for some serious "have you been a bad girl?" sexperiences.

DVDs. Buy a DVD on oral sex (check out recommendations in the Resources section), where you'll learn step-by-step how to assume oral sex positions, topped off with tips on technique. Not in the mood for instruction? Rent an X-rated film that's all about oral, or find an amateur download online. Either way, you have thousands to choose from!

Get creative. While there's always caution (and common sense) to be used in experimenting with items found around the house, look at the items you already have in your space. You may not necessarily have to shop at a sex toy store when you have things like a mirror in which to view your XXX-efforts. Or whip out your camcorder. Only instead of worrying about capturing the moment, have it there for her to appreciate the reflection of all the action in the lens.

Sexy Q & A

Should I be worried about her preferring these toys over my own equipment?

When it comes to a showdown between your penis versus a toy, know that a vibrator could never replace the thrilling feel of a hot, hard penis, for those who desire such, and that ladies are not always in the mood to jones their vulvas with vibes *au plastique*. So your fear of being bumped out of the picture is moot indeed. Both you and your partner should look at these objects as beneficial amplifiers and enhancements rather than threats to intimacy.

Sacred Oral Sex Approaches

It's time to take an "om" moment. After all, raw, unbridled sex can present itself in more ways than one, and ancient Eastern approaches to sex certainly,have a worldwide reputation for taking you to bliss and back. Stripping down to the core can make for some of your most unrestrained sexual pursuits and exhilarations, with sacred sex perhaps being the best vehicle for unleashing such. Sacred sex is an approach to lovemaking that seeks to join and celebrate lovers' bodies, minds, and souls. This spiritual discipline taps their sexual energy, which is seen as an embodiment of divine energy. This energy can be intensified and carried through the body via the breath, and other practices, setting every nerve ablaze. Sex is seen as a vehicle for enlightenment, a way to attain an altered state of cosmic unity.

The Allure of Sacred Sex

Realizing transcendence and oneness with your partner, nature, and a higher spirit is done over an extended period of time, with lovers riding a roller coaster of sexual response. It is during peak sexual activity, including extended orgasms, that lovers are launched into cosmic unity. While such can be experienced occasionally and spontaneously, it is with practice that lovers can consciously invite spiritual sexual union. This involves a tuning into your senses, harnessing your sensual, sexual energy, and living fully and presently in every moment.

Sacred sex has been practiced for over 5,000 years, stemming back to Hindu and Buddhist practices in India and Tibet. Best known in the form of Tantric sex, sacred sex is based on the belief system that a fusion of sexual energies is the union of each lover's masculine and feminine principles (yin and yang). Joining these opposite forces through lovemaking is seen as a way to achieving union with the Divine.

Sacred sex continually attracts lovers worldwide for not only promising personal and spiritual growth, but for holding the key to a more passionate sex life as well. Couples who practice sacred sex feel greater emotional balance, enhanced self-worth, and greater energy. The quality of their relationships improve, made only sweeter with ecstatic sexual experiences, longer sex sessions, and more powerful sexual reactions.

Rolls Off the Tongue

"We decided to take a sacred sex workshop, more for kicks than anything. But once we got into the practice, we were sold. It's no joke. Sacred sex has enhanced every aspect of lovemaking for us. With oral sex in particular, it feels more like a partner worship experience, with an emphasis on undying adoration and love." } Julian

| Oral Sex and the *Kama Sutra*

Written around A.D. 350, the *Kama Sutra* is the original, classic guide to extraordinary lovemaking. Written by the Indian philosopher Vatsyayana, this work was penned in an effort to help prevent divorce via good sex. After all, happy couples make for happy marriages. With oral sex in particular, Vatsyayana held that all sexual loving starts with kisses. This oral fixation is what sparks passion, sexual excitement, and the desire for more body touch. Lovers are to then work their way down from a partner's face, lips, throat, and chest to the arms, legs, and "joints of the thighs." The *Kama Sutra* encourages lovers to explore different kinds of kisses and ways each can arouse, with the nurturance of each kiss recognized as very pleasurable and reassuring.

An entire chapter of the *Kama Sutra* focuses on *auparishtaka*, the act known as "oral congress." *Oral congress* involves eight highly descriptive ways of performing fellatio, oral sex on a man. While progressive for its time, the work does note that oral congress is practiced primarily by gays, masseurs, and "unchaste, immoral" women. It actually gives hardly any attention to pleasuring a woman orally.

For our purposes, focus is given to what the *Kama Sutra* has to offer her oral pleasuring, as well as other tricks of the trade practiced by Tantric practitioners.

| Planning Your Sacred Seductions

Set the stage for sacred sex by creating a sensual environment. Influence the ambiance of your love chamber with happy pictures of the two of you, candles, bells, fruit, bowls, shells, plush pillows, oriental rugs, and tapestries.

In creating a sacred space, set up an altar in your bedroom or a special spot of your home that is only accessed by you and your lover. Decorate this members-only area with offerings, special items like candles, fresh flowers, and poetry. Include objects that represent her *yoni* (vulva), like almonds, fresh apricots, or triangles, as well as items that represent your own *lingam* (penis), like crystals and wands.

Add a final touch to your altar offering, placing a light stone on a dark velvet cushion or a dark stone on a light cushion. Stones to consider for their symbolism are the diamond for everlasting love; the ruby for a very deep, passionate love affair; pearls for long-lasting love; red jasper for warm, sensuous love; and garnet for sexual pleasure.

Finally, reconsider how your use of color, lighting, fabrics, and scents in the bedroom are (or aren't) creating a warm, harmonious, peaceful, and comfortable space. Hanging a violet silk, chiffon, or muslin fabric can invite female sexual energy, if so desired, while going for more red will stimulate your masculine vitality and life force.

| *Yoni* Kisses

While the *Kama Sutra* didn't say much about cunnilingus, a later Indian love manual, the *Ratiratnapradipika*, detailed the subject in the fifteenth century. Kissing the *yoni* (vulva) is said to symbolize reverence and respect for womanhood in Eastern cultures, acknowledging the role the female plays as giver of life. The *yoni* is cast as a flowering lotus, with the clitoris as its bud. Kissing and caressing her *yoni* releases sexual energy. And when her juices are flowing, and even ejaculated, the taste and smell of this sexual energy release are to be enjoyed.

Techniques for stimulating her *yoni* include the:

Pressing *Yoni* Kiss

Press your lips up against her labia, kissing, but not parting them. Make sure you're caressing other parts of her body as well.

Outer *Yoni* Tongue Strokes

Spread her *yoni* lips gently with your fingers and brush the outer vaginal lips with your lips and tongue.

Inner *Yoni* Tongue Strokes

Gently open her outer lips and brush the inner lips with your lips and tongue.

Kissing the *Yoni* Blossom

Spread her labia to expose the clitoris and lap upward along the shaft and across the head of the clitoris. Now lick upward along the sides of the clitoris.

Flutter of the Butterfly

Flutter the tip of your tongue along the clitoral shaft softly while kissing her *yoni*.

Sucking the *Yoni* Blossom

Take the clitoris into your mouth and suck gently, caressing it tenderly with your tongue.

Kiss of the Penetrating Tongue

Penetrate her *yoni* with your tongue, starting shallow and flicking entries and withdrawals. Move on to deeper tongue thrusts when desired.

Adhara-sphuritam ("the Quivering Kiss")

Squeeze her vaginal lips together gently and very slowly using only the delicate pads of your fingertips. Kiss the vaginal lips as though kissing her lower lip tenderly and tentatively.

Jihva-bhramanaka ("the Circling Tongue")

Use your nose to part her vaginal lips and open the vaginal canal. Insert your tongue delicately, taking your time to make slow circles with your face, allowing your nose, lips, and tongue to brush over and in her in circular motions.

Jihva-mardita ("the Tongue Massage")

Firmly slip your tongue inside her *yoni*, darting it in and out with gusto.

Chushita ("Sucked")

Press your mouth firmly against her vaginal lips and give them a deep kiss. Deliver gentle nibbles with your lips. Alternate lip kisses with a light sucking of the clitoris.

Uchchushita ("Sucked Up")

Lift her buttocks and as you're gripping them, put your fingertips in her tailbone indentations. Beginning at the navel, trace your tongue over her belly, giving light circular licks to the clitoris, then changing to big ice cream cone licks from the bottom of the vaginal opening to the clitoral hood.

Kshobhaka ("Stirring")

Open her thighs as wide as she can, then press your palms into her groin creases (if easier or more comfortable for her, she can hold her legs apart). Curl your tongue and play with her clitoris using rapid flicks.

Bahuchushita ("Sucked Hard")

On a couch, have her feet rest on your shoulders and hold her by the waist. Now bring her *yoni* to your mouth to suck hard on her clitoris with steady, lingering licks.

Sexy Q & A

Where does Taoism stand on the practice of cunnilingus?

Cunnilingus has traditionally been honored and respected by Taoists and is seen as a spiritually fulfilling practice that can increase the receiver's longevity. This is in part because ingesting vaginal secretions is believed to enable an individual to conserve and increase his or her *chi* (life energy) or vital breath. For over 2,500 years, this Chinese tradition has viewed female ejaculation, in particular, as sacred and essential to life. Her fluids are considered vital to both her and her partner and the cycle of life.

| The Crow, a.k.a. "69"

Referred to as *the crow, Kakila,* or *congress of crow,* the 69 position takes on great symbolism in the *Kama Sutra.* The Crow is seen as having great mystical powers, including the ability to dissolve substances, transforming original states into fusion form. In assuming 69, lovers are said to be "pecking" at each other's tender love parts like pecking crows, nibbling here and there, pleasing, and making delightful sounds like crows sometimes do. This kissing of the lower parts can employ any of the techniques mentioned in this chapter for sensation and pleasure.

Sex Savvy

Anoint one another. Honor your lover's body as a temple of your spirit by offering the body as a gift to the other and the universe. Mix an essential oil like rose with an oil base like pure vegetable oil. Then anoint each other's hearts with dabs of this concoction. Alternatively, you can mix sandalwood essential oil with an oil base and apply drops of this mixture to the area between your lover's eyebrows to awaken her Third Eye, the area between her eyebrows representing the sixth chakra (energy center).

CHAPTER 8

Owning Your Pleasures: Assessing Any Issues

You've gone from oral sex amateur to authority in acquiring and employing everything you need to know for the best this kind of sex play has to offer. Still, you may find yourself needing to perfect your pleasuring pursuits because it feels as though there's something wanting. In other cases, you—or your partner—may be fielding some issues that are trumping your game. This chapter is all about making sure that the two of you steer clear of anything that can throw your erotic efforts off course!

Common Mistakes People Make

Whether new to any type of sex or new to a partner, people will often need a few test runs before figuring out the right formula for flawless frolicking. Knowing which blunders to avoid ahead of time can have you presenting yourself as her best-ever right from the start. Here are the more common ways givers foil their own efforts.

You Don't Recognize the Need for Diversity

While there are generalities that can be made about human sexuality, the truth of the matter is that we're all very individual in our preferences, desires, wants, needs, and response. Every one of us is unique, sexually speaking, so realize that what might have worked for your last gal, isn't going to necessarily work for this one. You've got to approach a new partner as a clean slate, testing different moves and discovering what works (and doesn't) when it comes to upmost pleasuring. You've got to put aside any ego issues in the feedback she gives you as well. She's hopefully telling you what she likes and needs without sounding critical. Her being able to share in such a way should be seen as a compliment (in that she can be open with you) and not an indicator of something you're doing wrong.

Even after figuring out the right formula, you'll want to change up oral on occasion. Nothing spells sexual disaster like same old, same old. So consider novel ways to spice things up in keeping both of you interested in the oral action. Diversity is key.

You Ignore Her Other Hot Spots

It's easy to get lost in the focus of your attention, but your lover's body is covered with erogenous zones just dying for some equal attention. So don't ignore your lover's nipples, bum, or back of the knees, just to name a few of the favorite parts within arm's reach.

You're Not Easing Off the Clitoris

Every gal is different when it comes to how much stimulation her clitoris can handle, and this can vary from one sex session to the next. Sometimes, she may want it hard and direct. Other times, she may need you to ease off on her crown jewel, providing indirect or no stimulation. This can be in the very same oral sex session. So be sure to check in with her and to tune into verbal and nonverbal cues that she may need more or less of whatever you're doing.

You're Not Present

You had a tough day at work; you're feeling gassy from gorging yourself at dinner; you're wondering when you'll find the time tomorrow to pick up your dry cleaning. . . . There could be a million reasons why you're not into oral. But even if you're not into the moment, pretend that you are. Make sure that your hands are busy, exaggerate your head movements a tad, make some noise . . . pretty soon you may even start to believe your own performance and really get into everything you're doing.

She's Guilty of the Death Grip

While a squeeze of your head might seem like nice affirmation for a job well done, it's not. Amour needn't involve anaconda-like activities. Your ability to breathe is vital and only guarantees her continued bliss. For you guys who find yourself in this death grip, in getting some air without breaking up the action, grab her hands and squeeze them in yours, providing some much-needed relief for your head.

Rolls Off the Tongue

"It's flattering to know that she's totally getting off when she squeezes my head with her thighs, but come on! It hurts!" } Malcolm

The Need to Breathe

Drowning yourself in another's pleasure can be intoxicating. But it's anything but erotic when you have trouble surfacing for a little air. If you find yourself needing to catch your breath, some quick remedies to the situation include:

- Tilting your head slightly to the side to breathe through one nostril.
- Breathing through your nose, an effort made easier in staying above the sheets.
- Using your fingers while coming up for a breather.

There are also a couple of more advanced tactics you can employ in keeping your passageways open for easier air supply.

Circular Breathing

Circular breathing is an ancient technique which enables a wind instrumentalist to maintain airflow (and thus sound) through an instrument for a long period of time via inhalation through the nose. It's inhaling while you're exhaling, with the "exhale" based on your ability to fill the cheeks with air when you start to run low on the oxygen in your lungs and force it out as you inhale. It involves four stages:

1. As you become low on air, your cheeks puff.
2. Air from the cheeks gets pushed through the instrument, using your cheek muscles to maintain sound while you breathe through your nose.
3. As the air in the cheeks decreases, and sufficient air is inhaled into the lungs through your nose, the soft palate in the throat closes and air in the lungs is exhaled.
4. Your cheeks resume their normal position.

It is the switching back and forth from the air in the lungs to the air in the cheeks that enables a person to master circular breathing. Know that this doesn't come easily and does require practice. In mastering this effort, it is best to consult books and online resources, written by music instructors, offering circular breathing exercises. Need incentive? The world record for circular breathing runs at almost ninety minutes of continuous playing of a wind instrument. Now think about what that can do for your oral efforts.

Yawn

Open your throat muscles with a good yawn. Singers will often overcome throat tightness, especially in reaching high notes, by relaxing their strained throat muscles. So go ahead and yawn loudly. This not only allows your breathing to pass through without obstruction, it awakens you. Just be sure to explain to your lover what you're doing, lest you come off as being rude and bored!

| Common Concerns for Both Genders

Oral sex should be a stimulating, gratifying, amazing experience for men and women alike. But there are times where concerns can get in the way of one's ability to fully embrace oral eroticism. Here are just some of the issues that could be trumping your or your lover's game.

Self-Perceptions

"Am I doing it right?" "Am I good enough?" "Do I look ridiculous?" "How long until she reaches orgasm?" These are just some of the thoughts that can course through your mind as you're going down on your lady.

The solution: If you find yourself caught up in such worries, stop them and focus on the action, making a mental note to talk to your lover later in being reassured that none of these concerns are issues. Or you may just need some serious private reflection time with yourself, confronting the way you harshly judge yourself.

Guilty Blocks

Sadly enough, some lovers do not feel worthy of receiving affection. For whatever past reasons, she was made to feel that her sexual feelings, thoughts, and actions were wrong. Ultimately, her sense of well-being when intimate is compromised and she may be helpless to make the changes needed to overcome being her own worst enemy.

The solution: If this is your lover's story (or yours), consider consulting with a sex counselor or therapist in figuring out how to get to a better place and address what's needed from within, from your relationship, or from your partner in accepting the joys of oral sex.

Sex Savvy

It's just smart: Avoid oral sex if you feel ill, are drunk, or are high. Not only do these invite more of a gag reaction, they severely impact your sexual response.

Jaw and Tongue Fatigue

You're licking; you're sucking; you're flicking; you're massaging; you're tired. Whether tongue fatigue, neck pains, sore mouth, or the dreaded jaw lock, you're cramping up and are feeling like you've had your fill of a four star fine-dining experience. But there's a partner to be pleasured, and you want to be a trooper at this all-you-can-eat buffet.

The solution: Pursue any of the following:

- Practice jaw-strengthening exercises, e.g., chew gum regularly.
- Try using a different area of your tongue or let your lower lip take solo in providing stimulation.
- Pace yourself. Ideally, you'd be doing this to avoid the situation, but should it strike, resume a slow and steady pace.
- Carefully use your fingers to mimic your tongue until you feel recovered.
- Use Head Candy. This oral sex enhancement is candy pressed against your teeth to provide a soft, slippery cushion. It reduces jaw fatigue, protects your lover's loins from your teeth, and prevents dry mouth while increasing pleasure for the giver and receiver.

Just because you're dealing with mouth or body fatigue, doesn't mean you need to take a full time-out on her road to pleasure. Ways to maintain the action while taking a break include:

- Incorporating a vibrator to maintain hot-spot stimulation.
- Using your fingers.
- Mixing up techniques for variety.
- Changing rhythms.

Delightfully distracting her with some erotic talk or massaging motions over other parts of her body can further give you the excuse for a breather without blowing the moment.

Your Hesitancy in Being Submissive

Sex educators can't tell you how many times they've gotten the complaint: "He won't return the favor!" While they're all about being pleasured, some men can't get into a giver state of mind. The issue: You may think it's unmanly to perform oral sex on another. You may not like the idea of being submissive, feeling that it conflicts with your masculinity. While some men have been known to perform oral sex on call girls, they won't do so at home, feeling that giving oral to a woman is degrading to her. Complicating the issue even more is if you feel that oral sex is a sign that all of you isn't needed for pleasuring and satisfying your partner. You may worry that oral sex makes your penis obsolete. **The solution**: If any of this describes you, let your lover know your reservations. Expose yourself to sexually explicit materials that show mutual pleasuring, like the position 69, where lovers perform oral sex on each other at the same time. Be sure to highlight the greater pleasures and satisfaction that can be had in being a giver and receiving such adoration from your gal.

Sexy Q & A

Is it okay to kiss your lover after giving oral sex?

While some lovers have no problems with locking lips after oral sex, others will have nothing of it. Some people see this as a very intimate act and a testament to their bond in sharing everything, while others think it's gross, especially if emission was involved. To kiss or not to kiss post-oral really comes down to your and your partner's preferences. So be sure to talk about it and cases where it's hot versus not.

| Common Concerns for Her

A number of issues can prevent a woman from letting go and fully embracing her oral sex ambitions. Knowing some of the big trouble makers can help you work through her roadblocks of giving and receiving oral sex together.

Good Girls Don't

Feeling bad can feel oh so good, but getting oral might be pushing it for her. With so many women in our society raised to think that they shouldn't have sex until marriage, and that it should then only be "vanilla" sex (primarily missionary), it's hard for some gals to get past the negative messaging surrounding sexual pleasuring. A number have been taught that only "bad" girls do "sexplicit" things and that she's dirty and immoral if she takes part. She simply doesn't want that kind of reputation.

The solution: Work with her on examining the messages she has gotten about sex, including oral sex, over the years, tuning into how they make her feel. Are they fair or do either of you completely agree with them? Are they holding you two back from fully experiencing intimacy and getting in tune with your sexual selves, or are they completely justified? Challenge yourselves in determining if these are healthy messages or if there are other ways to look at sex acts that aren't so moralizing, demeaning, or sex negative. Make a list of the pros and cons of giving and receiving oral sex, educating yourselves about the physical and emotional pleasures and risks at play. You may just find that good girls "do" or at least try.

Rolls Off the Tongue

"It's so hard to know what's normal, especially when you might suspect something like a yeast infection. Nobody tells you what healthy discharge looks like.**"** }Sonia

Her Discharge

No matter where she's at in her menstrual cycle, a woman can stress over whether or not her discharge is healthy, especially when it isn't clear.

The solution: Get informed about healthy vaginal discharge, which can be clear and stretchy or "paste-like" and sticky, depending on where she's at in the menstrual cycle. Vaginal discharge can also be cloudy or whitish, turning yellowish when dried, and vary in volume, including when she's sexually aroused.

Sexy Q & A

Is it wrong to perform oral sex on a woman when she's menstruating?

If you want to have oral sex during the week of menstruation, talk about the potential in that with your partner. With a tampon or diaphragm in place, some lovers have no qualms with going down on a woman given there is no flow. Some aren't bothered in the slightest in coming in contact with her menstrual flow.

Your Stubble

She may love your beard or shadow, but not between her legs. Beard burn can be uncomfortable and hurt. So until you're clean-shaven, her legs will remain crossed.

The solution: Consider if a good shave would enhance your oral sex efforts. Then again, she may not be bothered by it. Ask her.

Rolls Off the Tongue

"I think the pain or pleasure factor of a beard comes down to the texture of a man's hair and how much hair he has. A friend of mine is totally not bothered by her husband's beard for any kind of fooling around. I, however, am not keen on it if my partner has facial hair, and would rather not be chafed, red, and sore between my legs the next day." } Laura

She Fears Losing Her Bladder

Related to feeling out of control is the issue of female ejaculation. This phenomenon is often mistaken for a woman losing her bladder. She may freak out in thinking that she has just peed during her orgasm.

The solution: Reassure her that female ejaculation is nothing to worry about. The fluid emitted when she ejaculates, mostly due to G-spot stimulation, only contains traces of components of urine. It's actually a prostatic-like fluid that's expelled into the urethral canal by the glands and ducts of the female prostate. Female ejaculation happens to some women some of the time when they are incredibly turned on. It—and the mess it can make—should be seen as super sexy reactions and nothing else.

Rolls Off the Tongue

"For the first time in my life, I felt embarrassed about my body in front of my most recent boyfriend. So I broke up with him; I hated being in a relationship where I was uncomfortable with being naked. Although I am a middle-aged woman with a less-than-perfect body, I know that I am beautiful for who I am and what I am. I don't think that he understood or appreciated that. It was important enough to me to end the relationship."

}Regina

She Fears Getting Naked

Inhibitions about her body and nudity can greatly impact her ability to be intimate with someone, let alone enjoy what's going on. These issues can creep up at any point in her life for a whole host of reasons, like weight gain, the appearance of cellulite, or a partner's negative reactions to her form.

The solution: The more reassurances you can give her about her figure and confirmation that it's perfectly normal and healthy to get naked, the better her ability to shed not only her inhibitions, but her clothes as well.

Rolls Off the Tongue

"I used to have issues with my body when it came to stripping down naked. I don't have huge boobs, and I have pretty wide, curvy hips and thighs, so I always thought I had the opposite of what men wanted. So I definitely never felt like a sexy woman. But then I was at a party one time and a guy—a famous rap star—said to me, 'You are sexy.' I was like, 'Huh? *Me*? Seriously?' And for some reason, that stuck in my head. Someone thought I was sexy. So, hey, maybe I was. From that day on, I decided I would start feeling sexier and amp up my confidence more. And the more confident I felt, the more people treated me like I was a sexy woman. And that translated into the bedroom." ⎫Sorah

Deeper Oral Sex Inhibitions

Whether as giver or receiver, people have lots of hang-ups about oral sex for a number of different reasons. In some cases, these can make it difficult for an individual to relax and let go and eventually experience the "big O." For others, inhibitions make for an oral phobia, with cunnilingus viewed as dirty, taboo, or a total turn-off. Some of these can be alleviated in getting to know your partner and feeling comfortable together. A supportive, healthy, loving relationship can do wonders for any oral sex issues. Yet regardless of one's relationship situation, there are situations that can lend themselves to a strong dislike or disgust of oral sex for men and women alike.

She's Worried about Losing Control of Her Entire Being

There's a great deal of vulnerability involved in having someone face to face with your groin, let alone making out with it, even when it's a most trusted source. It can be incredibly hard to relax and let yourself surrender to having your sexual response in the spotlight. She may fear making noise, getting too active, emitting fluid, or simply being the star of the show. This may stem from negative messages she received about sex growing up, messages she was taught about what it means to be feminine, or that she's not emotionally comfortable with the sex play at hand, her partner, or the relationship.

Rolls Off the Tongue

"I have to mentally give myself a pep talk when my lover goes down on me. I have to remind myself that it's okay to relax, forget about life, and just enjoy being pampered. Then I have to clear my head in tuning into my physical reactions and allowing myself to ride them to orgasm without any distractions." }Tina

Psychological Control

Sex is a head game more than anything, with your pleasuring boiling down to what's going on between your ears more than what's happening between her legs. Your mind can play games when it comes to oral efforts, especially if you've been raised with negative messages that oral sex is dirty or wrong, or you have trouble relinquishing control to a lover. Research has found, for example, that negative religious beliefs about oral sex restrain such sexual activity. Not being in a good or the "right" relationship can also get in the way of her being able to totally let go and enjoy the moment.

Reasons for the need to maintain psychological control during sex vary greatly, and may need to be explored with a certified sex therapist or counselor depending on her issues or yours. In the meantime, if either of your states of mind is controlling your ability to embrace oral, you need to learn to let go and replace negative thoughts with positive sexual affirmations. For example, she can replace an anti-oral thought with, "I deserve this kind of pleasure. It is wonderful and I will let myself succumb to it." Or in psyching yourself up to give, you can formulate a mantra for yourself, like "Oral sex is good for my mind, body, soul, and relationship. I will let it be so." Practice it on a regular basis.

Rolls Off the Tongue

"I remember something my brother once told me when I wasn't sure if a guy was the right guy for me. He said, 'Trust your body, your body knows if it is the right person.' I thought that was really interesting and actually found it to run true with me. Your body does seem to open up and do all the right things when it is the right person, but doesn't when it is the wrong person." }Preethi

Is "Third Base" "Real" Sex?

"I did not have sexual relations with that woman." Bill Clinton sparked a firestorm of furious debate in explaining his relationship with Monica Lewinsky with this statement. In many ways, the matter at the heart of the contested issue has never been laid to rest. Is oral sex "sex"?

For a few gals—depending on religious convictions or values they've been raised with around sexual intimacy—wondering whether or not oral sex breaks the rules can be very distressing. This can be complicated by social pressure they feel from others to put out. They just clamp up. In many cases, they just need to be presented with a safe space in which to analyze the matter for themselves.

As is the case with mutual masturbation and other sexual activities, many people don't see oral sex as "real" sex. It's getting to "third base," a step in sexual intimacy that used to be a big deal, but is now said to have become common as the good night kiss, at least among young people.

One Midwestern university study involving college students reported that the majority did not define oral sex as having "had sex." (In a similar vein, only 19 percent thought the same about anal sex.) Females were likelier than males to hold that fellatio and cunnilingus were not "sex." An earlier study by the Kinsey Institute found that while 99.5 percent of respondents held that intercourse is sex, only 40 percent saw oral sex as such. So what makes an oral sex act "sex" versus not?

This really boils down to personal opinion, and what a person stands to gain or lose in holding that oral sex is very much sex. After all, calling an oral exchange "sex" can impact one's virginity status, decide whether or not adultery took place, or influence one's perception of others, as well as the self. Research has found that a person's definition of sex changes based on the consequences involved in labeling an act "sex," and their perceptions of the sexual experience. Making matters all the more complicated is the fact that an individual's definition of sex is not always consistent with his own behaviors of what classifies as "sex" or not. The definition gets "tweaked" in an individual's hope to realize a positive result and advance his own interests, or, in the very least, not lose face.

Oral sex is likelier to be regarded as sex if it resulted in climax or if you're the receiver (versus giver). What a person is thinking about during sex and who you're talking to also influence one's willingness to see oral action as sex. A person's desire to expand his sexual resume, especially in making claim to "been there, done that" status, can impact his perceptions of oral classifying as sex. In clarifying what the oral action means to you and your partner, share your thoughts with your partner. This also helps the two of you to learn more about just how intimate this act is for either of you, whether with each other specifically or in the grander scheme of sex play generally (as people can have very different thoughts on the matter).

"There's no way that I'd ever call oral sex real 'sex' because my number of sex partners would sky-rocket. I've only had intercourse with a few people, but owning up to my oral quests would make me look like a real slut. I don't count those when I get asked about my number." } Chris

Sexual Abuse

It's very common for people—both men and women—who have been sexually violated to suffer from sexual repercussions later in life, though this is not the rule. Touch or certain sex acts can trigger memories and sensations resembling the abuse, stirring up feelings that majorly interfere with pleasure. Survivors may avoid or fear sex, see it as an obligation, experience negative feelings with touch, have trouble with arousal or feeling sensation, or feel distance or not be present, among a whole host of other difficulties. The after-effects of the trauma include fear, disempowerment, and distress, all of which shut down sexual response and interest. When sexual intimacy is managed, a survivor may experience numbness from unwanted touch. It's not uncommon for a person to avoid sex or see it as an obligation, which kills any enjoyment to be had.

In healing from this ultimate violation of trust, affection, and privacy, a survivor needs to seek therapy and sexual healing, which involves reconnecting with the body in positive ways. These activities involve couples receiving love, respect, and appreciation. This process of reclaiming one's sexuality as pleasurable and positive also involves introspective work, increased awareness of the self and body, developing positive attitudes towards sexuality, and acquiring new skills for touch and sexual sharing. It can take months or years, and is best done under the guidance of a counselor or therapist specializing in supporting survivors. This will require a great deal of patience for both of you, with the pleasures of oral sex to be had later versus sooner. Ultimately, both of you stand to reap the rewards in working through this healing process and the deeper understanding that can come out of it. Oral sex can be quite intimate, powerful, and incredible when it eventually happens.

| Overcoming Sexual Aversions to Oral Sex

An aversion is an unconscious, negative physiological and emotional reaction due to a person having had bad experiences with a behavior or extremely unpleasant emotional experience. A person with an aversion has learned to associate those bad experiences or feelings with a task or situation, and, hence, has been conditioned to react at the mere thought of these events with anxiety, distress, and unhappiness. Aversions can also stem from lovers trying to meet each other's emotional and sexual needs if this effort is associated with an unpleasant experience. These typically stem from a partner becoming physically and/or emotionally abusive, including putting pressure on a lover, or very sensitive when a need isn't met to his or her satisfaction.

Sexual aversion can reach the point that engaging in sex acts one wants to avoid can suppress sexual response or make arousal and orgasm unpleasant when they occur. Symptoms include a fear of engaging in sexual intimacy, attempts to make the sex act as short as possible, trying to find excuses to avoid or postpone sexual intimacy, feeling ill and/or depressed just before or after sex, and needing to build up your confidence before sexual activity just to get through it. The experience is more of a panic attack than anything, with some actually experiencing such during intimacy.

For you or your lover to overcome an aversion, you must break the association of sex with the unpleasant emotional reaction and associate it with a state of relaxation. This begins with learning how to relax when you think about sex. Set aside fifteen minutes a day to sit by yourself, be comfortable, and think about the experiences you have had. Notice the feelings that come up. Now, instead of thinking about sex, redirect your thoughts to relaxing experiences, making an attempt to relax different muscle groups in your body. Start from the feet and slowly work your way up, giving yourself time to unwind. Once relaxed, think about sex again, only stay totally relaxed. Don't think about the specific sex issue causing you distress, but imagine different aspects of sex, like your fantasies, noting your reactions. What acts hold appeal? Which ones do not? Remember to stay relaxed.

Write down what you learned about yourself. Which thoughts made it difficult versus easy to relax? Work through the ones causing you distress in future fifteen minute time-outs. Eventually, you'll want to learn how to relax at the thought of oral sex. Your goal is to stop the unpleasant reactions from occurring when presented with the situation. You can do this by relaxing at the thought of it, extinguishing the aversive association. Eventually, you'll want to relax yourself head to toe before an attempt to engage in oral sex. Note the feelings, relaxing your way through negative emotions that come up. These may prevent you from going all the way all at once and may take more than one attempt. Challenge yourself, but not to the point you're causing yourself distress. Once you have learned to relax at the thought of oral sex, see what you're capable of—and only after you and your partner have an understanding that you're the one in charge.

| How to Receive Pleasure

Whether overcoming sexual inhibitions or aversions, or simply wanting to improve your abilities to fully submerge yourselves in oral sex, there are some tricks of the trade you can both use to make every moment together more pleasurable.

Make Friends with Your Genitals

Don't be afraid to "own" your genitals. They're amazing and a part of you. So take the time to check them out, giving yourself positive affirmations for the sexual signature that is all yours. No two genitals are totally alike, and that uniqueness is part of the turn-on.

Pretend

Whether as giver or receiver, enjoy yourself, even if you have to fake it. Getting into the right frame of mind may be all you need in selling yourself on the act. You may even surprise yourself.

Masturbate

Become more comfortable with your sexual response and learn to turn yourself on—and become more orgasmic—via self-pleasuring. These private moments are vital in figuring out what works for you. This information can then be shared with your lover in maximizing the reactions to be had during oral exchanges.

Practice Your Kegels

Pelvic floor muscle exercises are well known for boosting your sexual responsiveness. This is in part because all of the major meridians that carry energy between the vital organs and body pass through the pelvic floor area in both sexes. Pelvic floor exercises help to strengthen the reproductive organs and the area's tendons. Exercising your PC muscle, as it's collectively known, increases blood in the groin, allowing for more sensations and reactions. So get started on a Kegel program.

Practice Patience

Guess what? She's not going to climax if she obsesses about reaching orgasm. Help her become less goal-oriented. In receiving pleasure to the fullest, encourage her to enjoy the ride and not worry about the destination. It's okay if there is no orgasm. It may or may not happen, and should not be seen as making or breaking an oral sex session. There are plenty of other factors to be enjoyed!

Health and Relationship Benefits

It's always good to know the health benefits to such sexual intimacy. These can themselves act as perfect excuses to lovers wanting to get it on, but feeling that they need a little permission to let go of inhibitions and oral away.

Sex, in general, is loaded with health and relationship benefits when your interactions with another are positive, informed, and healthy. And it's not simply the sexologists and health advocates hailing the wonders of sex. Even economists have claimed that regular sex can bring people as much happiness as would a $50,000/year raise. The more sex, it's said, the happier the individual.

Oral sex, in a safe context, can be a source of physical, psychological, and spiritual well-being. It can enhance your mind, body, and soul, offering:

- **Stress relief.** Being sexually active counters body tension, with sexual response releasing the cuddle hormone oxytocin into your system. Oxytocin stimulates feelings of warmth and relaxation, bolstering your ability to respond to stress.

- **Greater intimacy.** Oral sex can make for a stronger, longer-lasting relationship, enhancing the intimacy experienced between you and your partner.
- **Better sleep.** Sleep is the foundation of all health, with the orgasms attained from oral sex enabling you to catch some *zzzz*'s more easily.
- **Pick me ups.** Oral sex can boost your mood, with elevated arousal and orgasm-releasing, pleasure-inducing endorphins that can relieve depression and anxiety and up vitality.

It cannot be stated enough: Sexual fulfillment is a critical component of one's quality of life and health. Oral sex is one form of sexual intimacy that can help people to realize life to the fullest, making for more connected lovers and happier relationships.

Genital Perceptions: Attending to the Senses

She *so* longs to receive pleasure, but she has deep-seated concerns about her genitals. Trust me, she's not alone, though she'll feel like it. A number of people wonder if they're normal or if there's something wrong going on down there. People are reluctant to receive oral sex for a number of reasons, with lack of body confidence and knowledge about their genitals major barriers to such sexual pursuits. Many are worried about whether they smell or taste bad. Some fret over whether or not their genitals are unsightly. Some stress over the potential of performance issues, like problems with orgasmic response, given personal issues they have with what's between their legs. This is so unfortunate, because the attitude you have toward your genitals is an important component of your sexual experiences and your ability to let

Genital Perceptions

A study in the *Journal of Sex Research* reported that favorable perceptions of one's genitalia not only correlate positively with engaging in sexual activities, like oral sex, but enjoying such as well. How you feel about your private parts may, in fact, be more important than how you feel about your look overall. One study conducted at Old Dominion University found that perceptions of the body during sexual activity may be more influential on one's sexual functioning than the self-assessment of one's physical appearance.

Research in the *International Journal of Eating Disorders* further found that those satisfied with their bodies have greater confidence in their abilities to provide sexual pleasure to their partners. Lovers need to accept their genitals as a passion playground if they haven't already. Need more incentive? Individuals who are content with their bodies also report more sex and are likelier to attain orgasm.

Can your gal say that she has made friends with her genitals? Recent years have seen a lot of efforts focused on boosting female perceptions of their genitals, not nearly as much has been done for males. People are often really hard on themselves when it comes to what's below-the-belt, flustered that they don't look "perfect" down there. And they're not if they're comparing themselves to the altered and airbrushed visuals of waxed, makeup-covered, and even surgically manipulated genitalia portrayed in porn magazines and flicks. Ironically, nobody looks like those porn stars, including the models themselves. Yet many of us are guilty of holding everyone up to unrealistic, unattainable standards!

The Canadian magazine *See* reported that women who had viewed sexually explicit materials in magazines and movies admitted to finding themselves comparing their genitalia to the models featured, focusing on the "abnormalities" of their own genitals. This is critical given that research in the *Journal of Sex Research* has found that women who have experienced cunnilingus scored higher on self-rated bodily attractiveness measures than those who have never had somebody go down on them. Investigators concluded that the more people can see their bodies (and faces) as attractive, the better their sexual esteem and abilities to see themselves positively as sexual partners. So the key to your gal seeing the appeal in her genitals is realizing—and accepting—the fact that her look is what's normal for her. No two genitalia are alike, making your lover quite the awe-inspiring masterpiece to be worshipped with lucky you between her legs.

Rolls Off the Tongue

"When I first truly examined my vulva, I was struck by how one of my inner vaginal lips hung lower than the other. I didn't think it strange, since it has this flower petal effect. Just thought it gave my vulva character. With porn everywhere, it's hard not to compare, though. I never see models with vulvas like mine or those of other women for that matter. It can make you feel badly, but only if you let it. I've decided that there's nothing wrong with the way I look, and if anyone thinks otherwise, it's their problem." }Shakira

Her "Look"

It is rare to find a female with a perfectly symmetrical vulva. Yet, many women are confused over what's "normal" versus "ideal," going so far as to pursue tailor-made vaginas. Vaginal resculpting, costing thousands of dollars, may include labiaplasty (a nip and tuck of her inner and/or outer vaginal lips), vaginal liposuction (for a plumper, softer labia), and clitoral hood reduction (where skin tissue around the clitoris is trimmed). Yet the vast majority of women have unmatched inner labia, a clitoris that can be anywhere from small to large, and some degree of hair on her mons pubis, outer labia, and anal opening (at least prior to removal). This look is what is normal and natural for the female form and not what vaginal resculpting promises.

Judging Genitals

Adding insult to injury when it comes to the very personal matter of her groin: Some lovers have been known to judge a partner's genitals in not meeting unfair societal standards. Not knowing any better, they get turned off that their partners don't look like the latest *Penthouse* centerfold. Make it your mission to explore the vast array of vulvas out there, often found in educational human sexuality materials or being touted by sex-positive advocates like Betty Dodson.

It's important to remember that everyone is different and beautifully unique when it comes to what's between their legs. That's part of what makes every individual sexy and enticing. She needs to embrace what Mother Nature has given her! She needs to work on her self-confidence instead of trying to fix something that isn't broken. She needs to learn to love and appreciate the gems she has between her legs if she ever expects to awaken their full potential. The payoffs are huge!

So take the time to sit down with her and appreciate her body, getting to know what gives her genitals character and highlighting what you like about them. This could be her vulva's color, shape, folds, plumpness, protrusions. . . . Ask her to do the same for herself and for your parts. Remember, what's normal is to be different and your ability to respond sexually and experience and share pleasure has nothing to do with the way she looks, but how well she can embrace her sexual self in its entirety. Letting her know that you're perfectly happy with what she has is one way of supporting her in that.

Rolls Off the Tongue

"More than anything—guy or gal—I think it's important to look like you have a well-maintained bush. It doesn't matter how much or how little hair you have down there, just as long as it's clean and well-groomed."

}Kai

| Passion Amidst Pubic Hair

People sport all sorts of looks when it comes to their pubic hair, with color, amount, and texture varying greatly. Some go completely bare, while others strive for a specific style, e.g., the Brazilian, while others keep what Mother Nature gave them. For lovers pursuing passion amidst pubes, getting a hair stuck in your throat can happen, causing much discomfort and distress to those who have been there. So how do you avoid such? The easiest way involves combing through your lover's pubic hair with your fingers ahead of time. Massage her pubic area prior to going south as a part of foreplay, shaking loose any stragglers that could try to trump your game.

If the hair down there continues to be a problem, or if you're of the opinion that less is more, suggest hair removal as a form of foreplay or a sexy intimate session in and of itself. Lovers can spend a leisurely afternoon or evening together removing each other's hair, pampering each other with a sensual bath and erotic massage to boot. Hair removal can be as simple as a good trim of the hair covering the pubic bone, using manicuring scissors, to snipping the hair around or on the outer lips of her vulva to shaving, waxing, tweezing, or using depilatories along the bikini line. Lovers can have fun experimenting with different looks on occasion, and even color, given that, no matter what the form of hair removal, your pubes almost always grow back, albeit itchy and uncomfortable initially.

Smell: P.U. vs. Passion-Inducing

Every one of us has a distinctive signature scent, and we would perhaps do a better job embracing this natural aphrodisiac if it weren't for the smell-like-roses messaging we're bombarded with regularly. As you probably well know, sweating can cause a stronger genital odor. People can minimize unpleasant smells by avoiding synthetic (polyester) underwear, tights, pantyhose, and Spandex clothes that do not allow the genitals to breathe. Cotton underwear and exercise clothes, as well as loose clothes in general, are best in circulating air around the groin. Otherwise, bacteria can further set up shop, growing in a sweaty environment that causes undesirable odors.

The odor of one's sweat can also be influenced by diet, so be sure to avoid consuming too much sugar, caffeine, and alcohol, as these can make the genitals smelly. Do not use deodorants of any sort since these are not made for use on the mucous membranes of the genitals and may have chemicals that can irritate and cause an undesirable reaction.

Thanks to commercials, like those by Massengill and Summer's Eve, females in particular are brainwashed into thinking that they need to smell like morning dew or blossoms 24-7, lest they stink. If she's her own worst critic with her scent, it's time for a reality check. She needs to be realistic in her expectations. It's humanly impossible to always be shower fresh, but most givers prefer that their lovers maintain a certain level of cleanliness too. While people are not supposed to smell squeaky clean, humans are supposed to have a scent. So be sure to highlight the moments you think her genital region smells oh so good.

Her Scent

Every female has a vaginal odor of some type that is normal for her, with most women's smells often described as resembling plain yogurt, slightly pungent and sweet. The same bacteria (lactobacilli) actually exists in both environments, hence the common smell. This scent usually changes throughout her menstrual cycle as her hormones change, becoming stronger or milder. It is further influenced by her personal hygiene, diet, and genital health.

Her scent is perfectly natural and should not be considered a problem unless it suddenly becomes foul (e.g., fishy) or especially strong, which may indicate an infection (e.g., trichomoniasis or yeast infection) or another medical issue. If this is the case, she should visit her healthcare provider to determine the cause of the unusual odor.

Rolls Off the Tongue

"I think it's important to realize that even if I'm not particularly keen about my scent, a lover might be. After all, the smell of my genitals is supposed to be an attractant—and I've certainly had men say that it's an aphrodisiac. They love it and can't get enough of it. My attitude is: If a guy doesn't like the way I smell, maybe that's Mother Nature trying to tell both of us something, like maybe you're better matched with somebody else!" }Leslie

Scent and Pre-Oral Hygiene

Though smell-good products may sound like the perfect way to start an evening of oral pleasure, the vagina is self-cleaning and most products on the market are only going to upset the way her reproductive system regulates itself. Some of the products she should stay away from include:

Douching. Rinsing the vagina with water or a special solution (sprayed into the vaginal canal via a tube and nozzle) is not recommended. While women were once told that using a douche could minimize odors and wash away secretions, these products disrupt the vagina's ability to regulate itself. Douches wash away the healthy bacteria that line the vagina and alter the natural pH level of its mildly acidic environment. Douching can also spread vaginal infections to the fallopian tubes and uterus or lead to conditions like pelvic inflammatory disease (PID).

Vaginal Deodorants. These are unnecessary and contain chemicals that can irritate or damage vaginal tissues or the external genitalia.

Perfumed Soaps and Other Products. Deodorant soaps, bubble bath, and colored toilet paper are just a few of the whole host of products containing chemicals that can irritate the vagina and external genital area.

In staying clean while true to her natural smell, she should wash her vulva with warm water and a mild, unscented soap, like Cetaphil, Purpose, or Phisoderm, taking care to wash thoroughly between her inner and outer lips. Other safe, easy ways she can go into oral action feeling pristine include:

- Using baby wipes.
- Minimizing pubic hair so that it can't trap sweat and odors.
- Applying baby powder free of talc and cornstarch to the genitals.
- Spritzing no more than a few drops of a favorite fragrance near her pubic bone for a "European shower" effect.

Sex Savvy

A person's scent can impact whom we have sex with and how often. All indicators show that people are biologically programmed to prefer the scent of some possible lovers over others, especially when it comes to reproduction. With just one whiff of the skin's apocrine glands and the glandular secretion and flora present in the genitals and elsewhere, basic drives, feelings, and thoughts can be set in motion, with your nose letting you know you're aroused.

Sexy Q & A

Is it a good idea to have an enema before engaging in analingus?

An enema, or anal douche, flushes out the rectum, cleansing it of trace amounts of feces. Prior to rimming, some people use a mild enema, which involves releasing water into the anus to trigger a bowel movement or to rid the anal cavity of feces and bacteria. This is typically done two to three hours before analingus, as to give the body time to reabsorb the water before introducing the area to more activity. Over-the-counter disposable enemas are available at pharmacies.

When injecting liquid into the rectum and colon, use gentle products to avoid irritation or any cuts that could lead to infection. Enemas should also be performed infrequently since they may disrupt the body's eliminating process, as well as the rectum, bowels, and gastrointestinal tract.

Know that an enema does not treat or prevent the transmission of infections, including the spread of HIV. Regardless, prior to analingus, it's a good idea to wash the anal region with a moist, soft washcloth to clean the area as much as possible.

| Taste: Becoming a Fine-Dining Experience

In initially going down on somebody, unless you're using protection, your taste buds are likeliest to detect some degree of saltiness, though your lover may taste tangier or muskier at times. Her taste most often boils down to sweat and discharge, which is in part dependent upon her diet. Garlic and onions, for example, can result in strong odors that influence taste. Her taste can also come down to what you're used to and what you've been eating. Lovers who have diets high in soy sauce, for example, may not pick up on its influence on bodily fluids as much as those who use it on occasion.

In becoming scrumptious herself, your lady can pick out food to positively affect your experience. Encourage her to consume citrus fruits, like lemons, oranges, and grapefruits in sweetening her secretions. At the end of the day, you'll need to experiment with your diets to see how they affect your experience. This not only includes the foods and beverages themselves, but the amount consumed.

Exercise may also impact her taste, especially since we "sweat out" so much of our intake. If she's concerned about the way she tastes, she may want to taste her vaginal secretions the next time she masturbates or the two of you fool around (provided she's in good sexual health). Ultimately, however, just how yummy she is comes down to your palate, which you can't be faulted for.

| Be Supportive

No matter what her issue, it is one that she needs to feel able to overcome for better oral pleasing. Coming to appreciate her genitals and body is something she must do for herself—and her sexual enjoyment—and may require taking a human sexuality course or getting some sex counseling or therapy in dealing with any deep-seated issues. In the meantime, the best thing that you can do is to be a source of support, reassuring her about how much you love all of her body parts, and letting her know just how much you get off on pleasuring them—that it would mean a lot if she would allow herself to do the same.

Opening Your Mouth for Oral the Other Way: Sex Communication

Perhaps the next best thing to having oral sex is talking about it with somebody you like to orally adore. Sexy talk can be any kind of communication about sex, whether you're dealing with issues related to oral sex or discussing ways to change up or further eroticize going down on each other. Talking confidently is often what elevates the action to another level. Lovers in healthy relationships engage in sex talks that allow them to avoid or resolve sexual issues and relationship dilemmas, or take sexual experiences to a whole new level. Talking about likes, dislikes, fears, shames, fantasies, and emotional connection helps them to learn about their own and the other's beliefs, shaping their experiences

"In some ways, while the most difficult, our conversations about sex are the best ones we have because we try so hard to be effective communicators. This forces us to be more vulnerable in what we reveal and more careful with what we say. Even if we stumble, the extra effort we put into these talks highlights how much we care about each other." }Rae

| Talking about Oral Sex

For some people, talking about oral sex is a fairly easy endeavor. They can unabashedly discuss their desires, needs, feelings, and difficulties. They can also listen to such sharings without squirming. Yet being so sexually expressive and responsive isn't always easy. Most people aren't given opportunities to talk about their sexual beliefs, attitudes, and values in a safe space. Many people are not raised with healthy role models when it comes to good communication, let alone savvy sex communication. Making matters all the more difficult are negative reactions lovers can have when the topic of oral sex is touched upon. They're not only terribly uncomfortable, often becoming physically and emotionally withdrawn, but become critical, judgmental, and even verbally abusive in projecting their discomfort and upset.

It's important for lovers to share and ask about one's wants around oral sex, as well as any difficulties in giving or receiving. In having these conversations, lovers need to be mindful about keeping themselves in check, releasing any negative judgments and seeking to be patient with the self and others in overcoming any difficulties. Thankfully, there are rules of engagement that lovers can strive to abide by in making their efforts less stressful.

Rules of Engagement

In striving for respectful communication, it's important to realize that you're responsible for how you act and react. Take responsibility for your role, and have conversations marked by openness, acceptance, and appreciation; really listen for what's being said. With affection and compassion, reflect—and take steps—to make sure that it's understood. You can do this in making sure that the following guidelines steer your efforts:

- Have talks when you don't have to worry about any interruptions or distractions, and when you feel ready to give your undivided attention.
- Be sincere in stating your needs, wants, and limits, as this helps to cultivate your partner's sense of safety.
- Respect and support your lover, as this will help her to feel valued.
- Stay positive, avoid criticism, and think about what you're saying both verbally and nonverbally.
- Encourage more details with "Tell me more" or "I'm listening."
- Ask open-ended questions so that the response you get isn't so limited.

- Ask to take a break if you need one or ask if you can have some time to think about a matter before responding.
- Validate each other's feelings, e.g., "I didn't know that you felt that way. Let's figure out what we can do about that."
- Reflect on what you're thinking and how that's making you feel and react.
- Thank your partner for sharing, stating that you're glad that you talked if you feel that way.

Remember, it doesn't help to change the subject; to dismiss the other's fears, worries, and desires; or act like a know-it-all. Don't interrupt, use absolutes like "never," or use sarcastic, hostile tones. Finally, don't push your lover to the edge when it comes to oral sex expectations. Instead of getting turned on to your hopes, your lover will tune out. These sex talks can be intense, and you may have to have several of them on the same subject before feeling like you've made progress or fully shared and understood one another.

Initiating Oral Sex for the First Time

When you are initiating conversations about oral sex with a partner who hasn't been responsive to such sexual intimacy, request permission: Try "I've been thinking about oral sex and our sex life. Can we talk about it?" If she is unresponsive or dismissive, you can still state how this lack of reaction makes you feel and your concerns for how it reflects upon other issues in the relationship. If necessary, suggest that the two of you seek sex counseling or therapy, if simply for having a safe space, with a mediator, in which to air out issues. No matter where you have these sex talks, go into communication with no expectations, including thinking that you're going to change a partner's behaviors or attitudes. Your hope should be to simply feel heard, satisfied that you gave the chance at oral intimacy a fair shot.

Whether or not oral sex is ever realized, constructive conversations about this sexual behavior can result in greater understanding and emotional intimacy. Your hopes of being truly heard will be made more successful in making sure that your communication efforts involve:

- Listening, as well as paraphrasing and using reinforcement in reflecting what's being said. (Note: This doesn't mean that you are necessarily agreeing with your partner, but showing that you understand.)
- Being attentive by engaging and asking helpful questions to show you're into the conversation.
- Showing appreciation for what's being communicated, e.g., "I really appreciate that you're taking the time to work this out with me. . . "
- Showing that you value your partner, even when you beg to differ on a matter, e.g., "You know that I care about you a lot, but I'm bothered that you. . . "
- Using self-disclosure.
- Highlighting any positives about the situation.
- Encouraging more conversation, e.g., "Keep talking to me."
- Being physically supportive, e.g., holding your partner's hand.
- Owning your statements with "I" instead of other pronouns.

While sex conversations can be some of the hardest had, they're definitely amongst the most critical. The vulnerability and self-disclosure involved are intense, ultimately bringing lovers closer together and maximizing their pleasuring.

Your Nonverbals

While you've been giving a lot of attention to what comes out of your mouth (and your partner's), you also need to pay attention to the nonverbal messages you're sending to her when you're talking about oral sex. So evaluate your efforts revolving around the following:

- **Your eye contact.** Are you having trouble looking your partner directly in the eyes?
- **Body language.** Are you saying that you're open, or are your arms and/or legs crossed making you appear closed off?
- **Your facial expressions.** Do you look stone cold or are you being expressive in reflecting your internal reactions?
- **Your volume.** Are you getting louder, indicating that you're nervous or uneasy?

It can be hard to keep your nonverbals in check. And you certainly don't want such efforts to distract you from what you're verbally trying to express. But tune into yourself briefly, on occasion, to gauge if you would want to be talking to you right now, if you're somebody inviting more sharing in your nonverbals, and all of the other benefits that come along with that.

Who's Doing What?

There are times when one partner will want to take charge and please a lover to no end. Then there are times when sex is more mutually initiated, or, once the ball gets rolling, who is doing what orally will be decided in seconds. Typically, people see the giver as active, while the receiver as passive. At the same time, the giver is supposedly the submissive one, while the receiver is the dominant one. Yet there's a lot more fluidity in the power dynamic between roles.

In being a giver, you're very much in charge of the action. You're the one setting the pace, deciding upon the type of stimulation, and overall steering the pleasuring. For her as a receiver, she's very much in charge of her reactions. This involves her ability to let go and get out of her head and into the pleasure she's receiving. It also involves both of you being able to ask for what you want, provide direction when desired, and to give affirmations on a job well done. Unless couples are in a relationship where there's a major power divide between partners, or they're having fun engaging in such role-play scenarios, lovers are very much sharing the power dynamic for mutual pleasuring.

Regardless of your pleasure pursuit, the two of you need to be communicating about the kind of sex play you're after. Who will be the dominant and who will be the submissive needs to be negotiated, as well. Far from being tedious, the sex talk in and of itself can act as a form of foreplay, as you talk about how to make your fantasies a reality, and what it is about the scenario exactly that arouses you.

Rolls off the Tongue

"The action isn't always seamless as far as who is doing what, which is the only part of oral sex that was a turn-off. So we developed a signal. If I plan to go down on him, I draw a line down his treasure trail, and vice versa if he plans to go down on me. It's cute because sometimes there's a rush to be the first to make the line, while other times, we'll keep the foreplay going and totally tease each other in wondering who is going to make the line first. It's fun torture since that usually means that both of us really want to have the other go down!" }Celia

| Feedback

In striving to give the best oral sex ever, you need to ask for guidance from your gal. In some cases, your lover may be perfectly content, and honestly not have any guidance to give. In other cases—especially while in the moment and with new lovers—she will share quite willingly. So go ahead and ask about the type of motion preferred ("Do you like it when I move my tongue side to side or in circles?"). Ask what erogenous zones need to be touched more. Encourage her to tell you when to stop action, perhaps because a hot spot can't handle any more stimulation, and then when to start again.

In getting reactions from a receiver, your attitude should be one of "I want to learn and I long to please." Ask for information if it's needed ("Tell me about your _____") or tell your lover what needs to be done in order for you to maximize your efforts ("Spread your legs even more"). Or share what you're about to do or the reaction you're aiming for: "I'm going to make you. . . . " Go ahead and ask things like "What do you want me to do right now? Do you want me to go harder? Softer? Faster? Slower?" "What do you need for me to do more than anything?" "Does that excite you?"

In processing your oral sex experience or renewed efforts, ask each other:

- "What was that like for you?"
- "Was there anything you would've liked for me to have done differently?"
- "Where could I have given you more (attention, feedback . . .)?"
- "Based on what we just did, what would you like for us to do differently next time?"

Such guidance is almost always well received.

Sexy Q & A
How can you tell when a woman is about to orgasm?

You can't tell when a person is about to orgasm. While there are general sexual responses that most people experience as they approach peaking, there is no sure way to tell if your lover is about to climax. If you're concerned about your lover's level of satisfaction, ask!

| Keeping Oral Sex Sexy

Sex communication involves a lot more than talking about oral sex. It's also about those sensual, romantic, or really racy things lovers say as they're getting it on. Depending on the mood you're after or what the moment calls for, you can add to the other kind of "aural" sex by being:

- **Affectionate.** Let her know how much she means to you with "I love you" or "I adore being intimate with you."
- **Romantic.** Woo the giver with "You look gorgeous" or "The way you touch me when I _____ makes my heart skip a beat."
- **Sensual.** Ease the receiver with flattery like: "You smell amazing" or "You look so sexy" or "Your taste totally turns me on." "Your _____ feels so _____ against my lips."
- **Seductive.** Super-charge foreplay with statements like: "Love your _____ and I can't wait to _____." "I want to taste more of you." "I can't wait to feel you on my lips." "Does it make you hard when I lick you like this?" "Shall I continue?" "Ready for me to _____ you?"
- **Dirty.** Get raw and invite more XXX-action with lines like: "I want to feel it slide down my throat." "I want to lick you until it hurts."

If you're at a loss for words or don't feel like talking, keep in mind the power of sound. Moaning, groaning, gasping, screaming, sighing, wailing, whimpering, and crying for joy are all wonderful sounds people make in expressing pleasure and ecstasy. Likewise, moments of silence can allow lovers to enjoy their sex sounds, like heavy breathing, the wetness, and rustling of sheets. Tuning into these sounds during oral sex can enhance sensations even more.

Rolls Off the Tongue

"Having a lover who is good at aural sex can make all of the difference in the world. If somebody is going down on you, you can increase enthusiasm in doing things like talking dirty. If you're giving, talking sexy gives you the excuse for a breather, while not killing the moment." }Nate

| Talking about Safer Sex

Think oral sex is safer sex? Then you need to think again. As is the case with vaginal-penile and anal intercourse, engaging in cunnilingus poses sexual health risks which everyone needs to think twice about. Lovers need to take care of each other and their sexual and reproductive health in minimizing the risks involved in your oral fixation pursuits. It's not only the right thing to do, but can make everything even sweeter.

Sexually Transmitted Infections

Sexually transmitted diseases (STDs), a.k.a. sexually transmitted infections (STIs), pose some degree of risk any time anybody engages in unprotected oral sex. If one partner's bodily fluids are infected, he or she runs the risk of infecting another with STDs like HIV, hepatitis, syphilis, gonorrhea, chlamydia, and nongonoccocal urethritis, if semen (including pre-cum), vaginal fluid, blood, and/or breast milk are exchanged during oral sex or other types of sexual activities.

In other cases, STDs, like herpes, genital warts, scabies, and lice, may be transmitted simply via skin-to-skin contact. This is regardless of one's gender or sexual orientation. Confusing to many lovers is the matter of which STDs, like the herpes simplex virus strains, can be transferred from the mouth to the genitals and vice versa during oral sex. Infections, like thrush (yeast infection of the mouth), need to be of concern as well.

Sex Savvy

If both partners are infected with HSV-1 (oral herpes) and HSV-2 (genital herpes), they cannot re-infect one another or cause the other more outbreaks, including when one partner has an active sore or is experiencing viral shedding. This is because the body has developed antibodies to both strains of the virus.

Being knowledgeable about the risks of oral sex can only work to your benefit, making you a more empowered lover in all that you do, or choose not to do. With worries about your sexual health aside, you can allow yourself to get fully absorbed in the action. While a lot of what you're about to read may be hard to swallow (pun intended), you'll come away more sexually informed and sex savvier for it. It's hard to find thorough, accurate resources on this topic, so you only stand to heighten your bedroom rock star status in being completely in-the-know.

During oral–anal sex, you run the additional risk of acquiring hepatitis A, lice, scabies, anal herpes, anal warts (HPV), parasitic infections like amebiasis, and/or bacterial infections like e-coli. Kissing, licking, tonguing, or sucking on the anal opening with your lips and/or tongue invites the risk and spread of these harmful bacteria, viruses, and parasites, especially when exposed to anal cuts or tears or traces of bloody feces.

Rolls Off the Tongue

"I think I'd be more willing to give and receive oral sex if I felt more fully informed about the risks involved, as well as ways to protect myself. It's like people are afraid to talk about it because it's not sexy, which sounds ridiculous when you think of the consequences.**"** }Marty

| Factors That Increase Risk of Infection

In assessing the risk of acquiring an STD or passing one along, especially during unprotected oral sex, consider the following factors:

Active vs. Inactive Infection

While infections can be spread at any time, you want to avoid oral sex, or any kind of sex for that matter, when a partner has an outbreak, especially when either individual has open cuts or sores on or in the mouth or genitals.

Sex Savvy

A study of 300 people conducted by Johns Hopkins University found that the risk of throat cancer was nearly nine times greater for people reporting oral sex with more than six partners.

Oral Health

If you're the lover giving oral sex and have cuts, ulcers, bleeding gums, and sores in or around your mouth and throat, you're at increased risk of contracting an STD.

Dental Work

Related to your oral health is any recent dental work, including having undergone a root canal, having your wisdom teeth pulled, or getting dentures re-fitted. Going to the dentist for any kind of check-up or brushing or flossing your teeth before oral sexual activity also increases your risk of acquiring an STD. This is because these activities can result in lesions, scrapes, sores, irritations, or tiny cuts on the gums you may not even be aware of.

Sex Savvy

With early HIV research largely focusing on the anal sex practices of gay men, the scientific community failed to pay enough attention to the oral transmission of HIV. A presentation of eight HIV cases, given at the seventh Conference on Retroviruses and Opportunistic Infections, suggested that all of these eight cases were oral sex attributable, with all eight HIV-positive individuals having had some type of recent dental work.

Ejaculation

If your lover is performing oral sex on you and you ejaculate into her mouth, this increases her risk of infection. While it has yet to be confirmed, female ejaculation in one's mouth may also pose a threat.

STD Status

The presence of one STD increases the risk of acquiring another.

Sexy Q & A

When suffering from a sore throat and swollen glands, how does a person know if he or she might have an STD versus simply having the start of strep throat or the common cold?

There is no way to tell with certainty if you acquired an infection during oral sex or if you're coming down with strep or a cold since these conditions often share many of the same symptoms, like fever, swollen glands, sore throat, and tonsillitis. Indicators that you may have an oral STD specifically include oral lesions or cold sores, though this is not a hard-and-fast rule. Symptoms may also last longer than your average sore throat or cold. In determining whether or not you have an STD, or a more serious cold, pay a visit to a healthcare professional, who will take a throat culture to determine the cause.

When to Play vs. When to Abstain

If you or your partner have an active STD, it practically goes without saying that it's best to abstain from sexual activity until the infection is treated or goes back to an inactive status. If the STD is curable, make sure that you refrain from sex until treatment is complete. Be sure both you and your partner are tested and treated. Failure to do so could result in reinfection.

In cases where abstinence is out of the question or where a lover is carrying a lifelong, viral STD, safer sex options, as outlined in the next section, are available. You can further reduce the risk of transmission in having open, honest communication, limiting the number of sexual partners you have, and going for regular sexual and reproductive health check-ups.

All of these points are really important given that many STDs are *asymptomatic* (without symptoms). A person can be a carrier and never even know she is infected, especially since an infection may lie dormant in her system for months or even years after exposure. Thus, she may not be aware that she poses a threat to others. Take, for example, that two-thirds of the 45 million Americans with genital herpes never have any symptoms. Even when a person looks perfectly healthy, and the sexual exchange appears totally risk-free, make sure that you're both being attuned to the need to discuss and employ safer sex practices.

| Tools for Safer Oral Sex

Being on the birth control pill, or any other hormonal contraceptive, does not protect either of you from STDs, including HIV, during oral sex or other sexual activities.

The only way to protect yourself from STDs, other than abstaining from sexual activity, is to use a male condom, female condom, dental dam, latex gloves, and/or finger cots, depending on your sex acts of choice. No matter what your choice of protection, the key to avoiding infection is to use your prophylactic consistently and correctly. Latex offers the best protection, while polyurethane products are a great second choice for those with latex allergies. In any case, a non–animal-skin barrier should be used.

Here are prime ways to protect yourself and your lover during oral sex on her:

Dental Dams

A dental dam is a thin, square barrier, typically made out of latex, which provides protection against STDs, including HIV, during oral sex on a female and during analingus on any gender. It is placed over the body part you are stimulating on your gal. The Sheer Glyde dam has been approved by the FDA especially for safer sex. Other brands include Glyde Lollyes and Lixx.

At times hard to find, dental dams can be purchased at select drugstores or at specialty sex shops. Businesses specializing in safer sex supplies also carry dental dams in a variety of sizes. Many of these businesses offer confidential online shopping and shipping services for those longing to make discreet purchases. Certain sexual and reproductive health organizations, like Planned Parenthood, or your local Department of Health or campus student health services may also have them available for free.

If you have trouble finding dental dams, or are in immediate need of protection, there are a couple of around-the-house substitutes at your disposal. You can:

- Tear off a sheet of nonmicrowavable (since it's nonporous) plastic wrap, like Saran Wrap, for a thinner alternative.
- Using scissors, carefully cut off the tip of a nonlubed, "dry" latex condom, as well as its elastic band at the open end. You'll want to then cut across the length of the condom for a stretchable, rectangular barrier.
- Trim the fingers (but not the thumb) off of a powder-free latex glove and cut along the side opposite the thumb.

In using a dental dam, make sure you cover her entire vulval or anal opening area, holding the edges firmly with your hands as you feast away. For greater pleasuring for you, consider adding flavored lube to your side. In giving your partner more sensations, add a few dabs of your lover's favorite silicone- or water-based lube. When you've had your fun, be sure to throw away the dental dam since it should never be reused, shared, or reversed (or transferred from the vagina to the anus and vice versa).

Sex Savvy

Be cautious in performing oral sex if you have braces. First of all, you don't want to tear your prophylactic. Second, you don't want to draw blood. So be gentle, with both of you seeking to avoid sudden, jerky, or unexpected movements.

Latex Surgical Gloves

Whether you want to cover cuts on your hands or fingers, avoid jagged fingernails or hangnails, or simply want a smooth touch, gloves can provide feel-good sensations as you're delivering oral. Plus, they make for easy cleanup, enabling couples to seamlessly transition into afterplay and cuddling without worrying about mess. Nonlatex polyurethane gloves are available for those with a latex sensitivity or allergy.

Finger Cots

Found at your local pharmacy, these singular finger condoms are meant to protect fingers with cuts, allowing you to play with all sorts of parts while feeding your oral appetite.

| Talking about Your Sexual Health

Annually, 19 million Americans acquire an STD, which means that, sooner or later, you may have good reason to talk about your sexual health and safer sex with a sweetie. These discussions aren't easy, and if you're the one with an STD, you risk rejection, loss of confidentiality, potential humiliation, and other adverse consequences. Thankfully, there are ways you can prepare yourself for the tough conversation.

Get Informed

Knowledge is power, so become familiar with everything there is to know about STDs and safer sex. Educating yourself allows for greater understanding, ultimately reducing fears and giving you a sense of self and body ownership as you regain a sense of control and the power to cope. This also prepares you to correct any myths or calm any fears your lover may have.

Know Your Body

If you're infected with a viral STD, note when your outbreaks occur to better understand their timing. This might be when you're under a great deal of stress or drinking lots of caffeine. This will give you a greater sense of control over the infection and bodily changes, plus have you better able to counter triggers in taking better care of yourself and the best times to be sexually intimate.

Confide in a Professional

If you're distraught about your sexual health status or the risks involved in being intimate, talk to a mental health counselor.

Move the Conversation Forward Together

In successfully, confidently having sexual health discussions with your partner, be sure that they take place in an emotionally neutral environment and not when you're feeling horny and wanting to get all over her. Don't make a big deal out of them. This begins by not sounding anxious, panicky, or stressed rather seeking to sound calm and confident. You may also want to point out that STDs tend to get a bad rap. Oral herpes, genital herpes, shingles, and chicken pox, for example, are all due to having acquired a virus that remains in one's nervous system permanently. Yet genital herpes is stigmatized much more often than your common cold sore or chicken pox outbreak because it's related to sex.

Be open-minded and ask that your potential partner do the same. Discuss your levels of comfort with STDs and safer sex, weighing the risks in light of your relationship, values, and what's important to you in a sexual relationship.

Suggest that you put your heads together in crafting a game plan on how you'll protect yourselves from here on out, or at least initially. Some lovers may want to weigh the pros and cons of unprotected sex differently when in a long-term relationship, as some may be more willing to take or accept the risks involved in becoming more serious and intimate. In any case, tons of communication, trust, care, and protection are needed.

Talking isn't easy, but the benefits to your health and relationship are well worth it. Ultimately, you and your lover can feel closer in better knowing each other, and in becoming a team, protecting yourselves from here on out.

Sexy Q & A

What STDs are detectable even if you don't show any symptoms?

Both men and women can be tested for HIV, hepatitis, syphilis, chlamydia, and gonorrhea. Gonorrhea and chlamydia screening involves a urine test or swab of the inside of a female's cervix or the swab of the inside of the penis. Doctors test for syphilis using a blood sample or swab from a genital sore, if present. Blood samples are drawn to test for HIV and hepatitis. Unfortunately, no good screening test exists for herpes, though blisters or ulcers can be scraped for tissue samples. Women can have a Pap test done to test for an HPV infection. There is no screening test available for men in checking for HPV. Be sure to ask for STD testing specifically, as different doctors have their own agenda during exams and may not test for everything.

| Deciding Your Oral Sex Rules

New and different sexual relationships and opportunities require a constant re-evaluation of our sexual health, and just how much we want to or need to protect it. Ultimately, your sexual health comes down to your knowledge, skills, and motivation in protecting yourself. In becoming more informed, you learn more about your choices. You can do what's best for you given how much you're willing to roll the dice—or not.

So take the time to assess your levels of risk and decide upon the rules that will guide your oral sex efforts. You may, for example, always require a barrier method when having oral sex with somebody you just met. You may require that a partner get tested before having unprotected oral sex. This is a game where you draft your own guidelines, and hopefully have a partner who is on the same page.

CHAPTER 11

Maximizing Her Orgasmic Potential

When it comes to sexual intimacy, nothing is quite as coveted as having an orgasm. Lovers spend a lot of time experimenting with different ways to reach climax, playing with the various hot spots sprinkled on or inside the body. With no two orgasmic experiences alike, lovers can elicit all sorts of climaxes and other reactions from one sex session to the next. Maximizing these during oral sex only adds to the infatuation lovers have with the pleasures had during such intimate exchanges.

"I think that one of the reasons going down on a woman is the best is because they're so orgasmic from it. I get so caught up in her pleasure, and I know that I'm a huge reason why she's in ecstasy. I've often had to reassure girlfriends that I love it, and then once they let me and realize that I'm all about it, they keep coming back for more!" }Bennett

| Oral Orgasms for Her

For some women, oral sex is the only way to reach orgasm or experience multiple orgasms. This is in large part because a woman's clitoris gets so much attention. Playing with this hot spot is vital to her orgasmic response, with over 70 percent of women needing clitoral stimulation in order to peak during any type of sexual activity. According to the *Hite Report*, 42 percent of women regularly climax during oral stimulation. And the *Janus Report* revealed that 18 percent of women reported preferring orgasm from oral sex than intercourse.

Rolls Off the Tongue

"The best orgasms come when your efforts are geared to your partner having the best orgasms. It's a spiritual event." }Tiffanie

Multiple Orgasms

For some women sexual response induced from oral sex may result in multiple orgasms. Such a climactic response may present itself generally in any of the three following ways:

- **Compound single orgasm.** Each climax occurs separately, with an individual going back to a semi-aroused state between these peak responses, e.g., having a second orgasm a half an hour later.

- **Sequential multiple orgasms.** Involves a series of climaxes that happen anywhere from two to ten minutes apart. Re-stimulation may be necessary.
- **Serial multiple orgasms.** These orgasms occur in succession, with one right after the other. They may be separated by seconds. In other cases, these orgasms can feel like one huge, long orgasm. In either case, she may feel as though she is riding wave after wave of pleasure.

One of the ways people experience an orgasm or multiple orgasms during oral sex is in the giver's ability to maintain a steady, constant rhythm when it comes to the action. In some cases, more pressure or a faster pace may be necessary. In any case, the giver needs to maintain action in seeing the receiver's response through to orgasm.

Sexy Q & A

What are other types of orgasm a female can experience besides the clitoral, G-spot, and blended?

While a female may not experience every kind of orgasm to be had, every female has the potential to experience them, including:

- **Nocturnal.** Like males, she can experience "wet dreams" when she sleeps.
- **Cervical.** This orgasm is triggered by stimulation of her cervix.
- **Nipple.** Playing with her breasts and nipples can invite climax.
- **Anal.** Stimulation of the anus or anal opening can result in this type of orgasm.
- **Spontaneous.** These "extragenital orgasms" are due to erotic thoughts, including from "thinking off," or triggered when a part of her body is touched during daily activities, e.g., while doing sit-ups.

Simultaneous Orgasms

Simultaneous orgasm is where lovers experience climax at the same time. While this can take place at any point during oral sex, depending on how you are being stimulated (including mentally), realizing simultaneous orgasm is often desired during 69. Engaging in *soixante-neuf* can elicit orgasm at the same time for lovers, provided that your sexual response states are in-sync.

While fun, lovers should be wary of making simultaneous orgasm the goal of sex since it tends to be the exception, not the rule. It's also quite sweet and sensuous to see a lover climax instead of necessarily being caught up in your own at the exact same time.

Rolls Off the Tongue

"We get lucky with simultaneous orgasm on occasion during 69, but in some ways it's more fun to take turns. It can be hard to really enjoy your own orgasm and somebody else's at the same time, so we tend not to make it our focus." }Frederick

| Incorporating Other Hot Spots

While clitoral stimulation certainly makes for orgasmic reactions during oral sex, playing with other hot spots in addition to the oral action can make for different types of orgasms. No matter what you do, make sure you're communicating with the lady being attended to. What does she like? Dislike? Need more or less of? The clitoris is a wonderfully hot spot that can at times, and for some more than others, be too much of a good thing, so make sure that she's totally comfortable. And if she needs a breather, don't take offense. Take it as a compliment!

Her G-Spot

Playing with the G-spot and a woman's clitoris during oral sex can result in a blended orgasm, where both her pudendal and pelvic nerves are triggered for an even stronger orgasmic response. Women have described these types of orgasms as deeper both physically and emotionally, and ultimately more satisfying.

To stimulate her G-spot, make sure that she's aroused. Then, using two or three well-lubed fingers, feel for a swollen, puckered, wrinkly area along the front wall of the vagina. Once found, stroke this area firmly and rhythmically, checking in with her as to what feels good (or not). Slowly increase the rhythm, adding pressure for more friction. Continue this action as you begin to pleasure her clitoris with your tongue and lips. For variety, thrust your fingers in and out of her vagina, "bumping" up against the G-spot. Or try rhythmically sliding or rocking your fingers across this hot spot in working her to the "big O." For smoother execution, try keeping your mouth/tongue and hand action in rhythm.

Her Bum

For a number of people, the bum is a hot spot in and of itself. She may just love having you grab, spank, or pull on her meaty, curvy buns as you enjoy the moment. You can also massage or grip her butt cheeks while giving head, pinching, or digging your nails into them in letting her know how turned on you are. Taking hold of her bum also allows you to better direct the angle, speed, and depth of the action. So don't be afraid to take charge!

Regardless of what you choose to do, the natural giggles that result will have a ripple effect throughout her loins, with her nerve endings in full effect from a tickling or light stinging you've managed. Make these areas ache even more in toying with her butt crack, running your fingers (or tongue during analingus) up and down the crease for greater stimulation. In making your fingers more of a gliding movement, use some lube.

Her Anus

Even if she's turned off to anal penetration of any sort, that's not to say that she may not be up for a little action around the anal opening. The external opening is an area that's full of sensitive—and responsive—nerve endings which fire up when she becomes sexually excited. This area may come to life as more blood fills the area, making her more aroused and sensitive to your efforts. She may also get off on the taboo element of it.

One thing to realize when it comes to anal play is that the area needs to be seduced. You don't just want to rush in; rather the anal area needs a little bit of foreplay itself if it is to be fully enjoyed. Most lovers don't like to be taken by surprise, so slowly work your fingers or tongue to the area. See analingus as one leisurely way to warm up her engines, slowly working your way to French kissing the area for her enjoyment.

| Tips for Maximizing Her Orgasmic Response

Sometimes you may want to further intensify sex sessions. Other times, you may need to employ a few tricks in evoking more of an orgasmic response, especially during hot spot play that isn't working the way you want it to. In inviting more of a reaction, try the following.

Have Her Get out of Her Head

Explain to her that she doesn't always need to be in control. Instead of resisting her sexual response, be a catalyst and relax, giving into sensations and the joy of being pleasured. She needs to get into the same head space as she would be in going for a deep tissue massage. She's here to take care of herself, let you do the work for her, and not think, but enjoy and lose herself in the feel-good sensations!

Teach Her Relaxation Exercises

If she's obviously stressed about receiving oral or is having trouble letting go for a more orgasmic response, guide her in the process of becoming more centered in her body. The following slow, conscious breathing exercises will help to reduce her stress levels and to enhance her sexual awareness and sexual focus, while bringing her back to or into her body. Encourage her to take deep inhalations that fill her belly. She should strive to widen her ribcage and lift her chest with the inhale. On the exhale, she wants to make throaty sighs to relax the body. These not only sound sexy, but make her more receptive to pleasure.

You can also instruct her to consciously send warmth to a part of her body, directing her focus to an area. She should then focus on the warmth, sending breaths to the area.

Encourage Her to Get Active

Sometimes she needs to move and get into the action, especially when it starts to feel divine. So have her get that pelvis of hers moving. Encourage her to squeeze her pelvic floor muscles rhythmically with your tongue movements or the sucking or thrusting action. Ask her to stimulate hot spots that you're unable to attend to. While sometimes it's nice to lay there, other times you may need to get more physically responsive.

Fantasize

Give her your blessing to lose herself in a favorite fantasy or pretend that the situation is slightly different than what it is. This may be imagining that you are her favorite movie star. This could be envisioning that she's the star of a sold out sex show. She needs to think about what may be more desirable when it comes to the who (sorry, but it's often so), what, when, where, and why for a completely different sexual situation that could throw her over the edge.

Get a Little Help

Whether either of you is tired, or she's not reacting in the way you hoped, whip out a favorite vibrator and let it do all of the work. After all, these toys are there to enhance, help you out, and bring on reactions otherwise oft unattainable.

Tease

While it's good to have great sexpectations, knowing what's going to happen can make for monotonous instead of moan-worthy action. So tease your lover, building sexual tension as you take her to the edge of bliss, only to attend to another hot spot. Keep coming back to her clitoris, but back off until neither of you can bear it anymore. Then relish basking in a state of maximum sexual response.

Rolls Off the Tongue

"I love both giving and receiving, but there's something about my partner becoming putty in my hands when I'm the one delivering. When I love and care about the person, it's so gratifying to know that they're feeling good and that my tongue and lips were the main cause for that!"

}Richard

Make Sure You Get Some Too!

Everybody has personal preferences when it comes to being giver or receiver. Ideally, there are times you want to give, and then there are times you want to receive. And research shows that people are fairly good at taking turns: 77 percent of men and 68 percent of women have given oral sex to a partner, and 79 percent of men and 73 percent of women have received oral sex from a partner.

Unless lovers have absolutely no qualms about it, one-sided oral sex always raises red flags. Not only is it a reflection of the quality of intimacy, namely the level of detachment, in the relationship, but it speaks volumes as to the lack of concern for mutual pleasuring. Even in cases where a lover feels all-powerful in seducing another in an effort to show off how good they are at giving, there's a certain level of exploitation when one partner is always servicing the other. To make sure she's comfortable satisfying you in the same way, make sure you understand the facts in play on her side of things.

- In general, research has found that a greater proportion of women enjoy receiving more than giving. Only a small percentage of women say that they thoroughly enjoyed giving.
- A major motive in giving oral for both sexes is to "return the favor." This expectation plays heavily in a person's willingness to go south of the border. Whether or not they plan to reciprocate, some people feel uncomfortable at the mere thought that they're expected to return. Typically, women report feeling obliged to give head to a partner after he went down on them.
- While your decision to go down on her supports your belief in your sexual prowess and competency as a lover, her main motive to give head may simply be to please you—not herself.
- The same concerns that could keep her from enjoying the oral sex you offer, could be standing in the way of giving you oral sex, too.

Ultimately, it's important to communicate your needs and desires with her. The best types of oral sexual experiences involve mutual pleasuring. While one sex session doesn't have to involve each partner receiving, lovers in healthy relationships tend to make sure that each has their time in the limelight. This is regardless of one's level of enthusiasm in wanting to give, or not. After all, in wanting to make a lover happy, in longing to rock his or her world to the core. Making this attitude one of 50-50 is key.

Obviously, you're a giver. You just read an entire book on how to give her some of the best oral sex ever. If being a pleaser is in your nature, especially when it comes to sexual exchanges, it can be hard to let your lover do all of the "work." But rest assured, most lovers will be more than willing to let you have your turn. Realize, too, that it is sometimes better to give than to receive and that your actually allowing your partner to feel pleasure in pleasing you.

So give yourself permission to relax and be receptive. Mutual pleasuring is a must for a thriving, satisfying sex life, and your ability to invite such will make oral sex better for both of you no matter what your roles.

APPENDIX A

Glossary

69 see "Sixty-Nine."

Afterplay post-sex touch and play.

Anal Beads plastic or latex beads strung together on a nylon or cotton cord that are used for anal sex play.

Anal Intercourse a sexual behavior involving insertion of one person's penis into another's anus.

Analingus stimulation of the anus with the mouth.

Anus the rectal opening located between the buttocks.

Bartholin's Glands two small glands, just inside the inner lips of the vagina, which secrete a small amount of fluid during sexual stimulation, a.k.a. "Greater Vestibular Glands."

Ben Wa Balls small, solid metal balls inserted into the vagina for sexual stimulation.

Butt Plug a dildo specially designed for anal and rectal pleasure via insertion into the anus.

Cervix opening to the lower part of uterus which protudes into the vagina.

Clitoral Hood a sheath of tissue which protects the clitoris and is an extension of the inner lips that run alongside the vaginal opening.

Clitoris the female's highly sensitive sexual organ, located in front of the vaginal entrance and urethra, that is filled with a high number of nerve endings.

Cunnilingus stimulation of the female genitals with the mouth.

Dental Dams latex or plastic wrap barriers placed over the vagina or anus during sexual activity to prevent the spread of STIs.

Dildo an artificial penis made of rubber, silicone, or latex.

Female Condom a disposable, polyurethane contraceptive tube, with a plastic ring at each end, that is inserted into the vagina to prevent pregnancy and the transmission of STIs and HIV.

G-spot small mass of erectile nerve tissue, ducts, glands, and blood vessels located between the pubic bone and the front of the cervix.

Inner Lips see "Labia Minora."

Labia Majora rounded pads of fatty and fibrous tissue, covered with pubic hair, that lie on either side of the vaginal entrance.

Labia Minora thin folds of skin that lie on either side of the vaginal entrance and extend forward to come together in front of the clitoris to form the clitoral hood.

Mons Pubis the fatty pad of tissue and skin under a woman's pubic hair, over her pubic bone, which is thought to protect her pubic bone from damage during vigorous sexual thrusting.

Multiple Orgasms a series of orgasmic responses that generally occur without dropping below the Plateau Level of arousal.

Oral Sex sexual activity involving mouth stimulation of the genitals.

Orgasm series of involuntary muscular contractions and a feeling of intense pleasure focused in the genitals that peak at sexual arousal and that may spread throughout the body; third and shortest phase of the sexual response cycle.

Rimming see "Analingus."

Safer Sex vaginal, anal, or oral sex involving practices that reduce the risk of pregnancy, HIV, and STIs.

Sexually Transmitted Disease (STD see "Sexually Transmitted Infection."

Sexually Transmitted Infection (STI any disease that can be transmitted via sexual contact.

Sixty-Nine stimulation of the genitals with the mouth by both partners at the same time.

Soixante-Neuf see "Sixty-Nine."

STD see "Sexually Transmitted Disease."

STI see "Sexually Transmitted Infection."

Urethral Opening an acorn-shaped protrusion found between the clitoris and vaginal opening, through which urine passes.

Vagina highly muscular, three-to-four–inch-long, tube-shaped organ in the female, which the penis is inserted into during sex, and through which a baby passes during birth.

Vaginal Opening entrance leading to the female's vagina, through which a baby passes during birth and through which menstrual blood passes during her period.

Vibrator a battery-operated or electric device that vibrates to stimulate body parts, particularly the genitals.

Vulva a collective term for the female external genitals: the clitoris, mons pubis, inner lips, outer lips, labia majora, urethral opening, and vaginal opening.

APPENDIX B

Resources

Internet Resources

American Social Health Association

www.ashastd.org

Offers sexual health information, particularly on sexually transmitted infections.

Centers for Disease Control and Prevention

www.cdc.gov

Presents sexual and reproductive health information. Oral sex and HIV risk information can be found at: *www.cdc.gov/hiv/resources/factsheets/pdf/oralsex.pdf.*

Go Ask Alice!

www.goaskalice.columbia.edu

Columbia University's Health Education Program Q&A site.

Sexuality Information & Education Council of the United States

www.siecus.org

A nonprofit organization providing sex education programs and materials.

Sexuality Source, Inc.

www.sexualitysource.com

Offers sex education and consulting services, plus sex coaching information at *www.sensualfusion.com.*

| Additional Reading

Female Ejaculation

Female Ejaculation & the G-spot by Deborah Sundahl (Hunter House, 2003). Alameda, CA.

Unlocking the Secrets of the G-Spot Video. (DVD). (Sinclair, 2000).

Fantasy

The Erotic Guide to Sexual Fantasies for Lovers. (DVD). (Sinclair).

G-Spot

Maximizing G-Spot Pleasures. (DVD). (Sinclair).

Whipple, Dr. Beverly, John D. Perry, and Alice Khan Ladas. *The G-Spot and Other Discoveries about Human Sexuality.* (Holt Paperbacks, 2004). New York, NY.

Kama Sutra

The Better Sex Guide to the Kama Sutra Set. (DVD). (Sinclair, 2004).

Sex Communication

Fulbright, Yvonne K. *Sultry Sex Talk to Seduce Any Lover: Lust-Inducing Lingo and Titillating Tactics for Maximizing Your Pleasure.* (Quiver, 2010). Beverly, MA.

Sex Therapy

American Association of Sex Educators, Counselors & Therapists

www.aasect.org

Society for Sex Therapy & Research

www.sstarnet.org

Sex Toys and Sexual Enhancements

Babeland

www.babeland.com

Sinclair Intimacy Institute

www.sinclair.com

Sexual Health

Fulbright, Yvonne K. *The Hot Guide to Safer Sex.* (Hunter House, 2003). Alameda, CA)

Planned Parenthood Federation of America

www.ppfa.org

Sexual Health Network

www.sexualhealth.com

Provides sexuality information, education, and other resources.

Sexual Pleasuring

Chalker, Rebecca. *The Clitoral Truth: The Secret World at Your Fingertips.* (Seven Stories Press, 2000). New York, NY.

Fulbright, Yvonne K. *The Better Sex Guide to Extraordinary Lovemaking.* (Quiver, 2010). Beverly, MA.

——. *Pleasuring: The Secrets to Sexual Satisfaction.* (Hollan, 2008). Beverly, MA.

——. *Touch Me There! A Hands-On Guide to Your Orgasmic Hot Spots.* (Hunter House, 2005). Alameda, CA.

Stewart, Jessica. *The Complete Manual of Sexual Positions.* (Sexual Enrichment Series). Chatsworth, CA.

Tantric Sex

Anand, Margo. *The Art of Sexual Ecstasy.* (Putnam, 1989). New York, NY.

Lacroix, Nitya. *The Art of Tantric Sex.* (DK, 1997). New York, NY.

Sarita, Ma Ananda and Swami Anand Geho. *Tantric Love.* (Fireside, 2001). New York, NY.

Schulte, Christa. *Tantric Sex for Women.* (Hunter House, 2005). Alameda, CA.

Oral Sex Instructional DVDs

Better Sex Video Series: The Art of Oral Loving. (DVD). (Sinclair, 2006).

The Expert Guide to Oral Sex Part I: Cunnilingus. (DVD). (Tristan Taormino, 2006).

Nina Hartley's Advanced Guide to Oral Sex. (DVD). (Adam & Eve, 1998).

Index

Note: Page numbers in *italics* include illustrations.

Confidence
> body issues and, 102
> enthusiasm and, 60
> genital perceptions and, 114, 116
> sexual aversions and, 107
> in sexual health discussions, 143
> taking charge with, 48

Congress of crow. *See* 69 position

Control issues, 102–4

Crow position, 89

Cunnilingus. *See also* Fellatio
> definition of, 2
> education and, 7
> illegality of, 4
> Napoleon and, 9
> safety of, 134
> taboo of, 102
> Taoism and, 89
> using Altoids during, 74

Cushions, 27, 81, 86

Dental dam, 74, 139–41

Dental work, 137

Deodorants, vaginal, 120

Desire, 16, 17–18

Dildos, *78*

Discharge, 99–100

Diversity, 92

Dopamine, 44

Douching, 120, 121

DVDs, 82

Eating ass. *See* Analingus

Eating someone out. *See* Cunnilingus

Ejaculation, female
> definition of, 19–20
> infections from, 137
> sacred, 89
> understanding, 101

Endorphins, 75, 111

Enemas, 121–22

Erogenous zones. *See also* Hot spots
> after orgasms, 92
> feedback on, 132
> G-spot as, 16
> labia as, 13
> massaging, 49
> shower spray on, 51
> targeting, 9
> types of, 92
> using mouth on, 59
> vibrators for, 78

Fantasies, 54, 151–52

Feedback. *See* Communication

Fellatio, 85, 105. *See also* Cunnilingus

Finger(s)
> *Adhara-sphuritam* and, 88
> in anus, 67, 150
> breathing and, 94
> on clitoris, 60, 63, 64
> cots, 139, 141
> on erogenous zones, 49
> fatigue and, 97

About the Author

Yvonne K. Fulbright, PhD—sexologist, author, relationship expert, advice columnist, and television and radio personality—has been featured in hundreds of media outlets around the globe, including Fox's *Red Eye, USA Today,* the *New York Times, Men's Health UK,* and the Austrian Broadcasting Company. Yvonne received her master's degree in human sexuality education from the University of Pennsylvania and her PhD in international community health education, focusing on sexual health, from New York University. She is currently a professor at both American University and Argosy University, the sex columnist for *Cosmopolitan* and Iceland's *Morgunbladid,* and resident sexual health and relationship ambassador for Astroglide. Yvonne also blogs for Huffingtonpost.com and is the sex expert for Comcast's "Dating on Demand" squad, SexHealthGuru.com, cherrytv.com, and the syndicated radio show *Your Time with Kim Iverson.* She is a Certified Sex Educator through the American Association of Sex Educators, Counselors, and Therapists (AASECT), where she provides editorial direction for *Contemporary Sexuality.* Yvonne currently lives in Washington, D.C., where she runs SensualFusion.com. For more information on Yvonne, visit *www.sexualitysource.com.*